FRIEND
Biotech

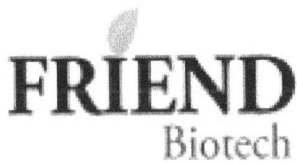

THE LINK BETWEEN
NUTRITION
GLUTATHIONE
AND
COVID-19

What they may not have told you

LEE FRIEND

Version - Draft 15.6

www.friendbiotech.com

Please note that the author is a researcher specialising in amino acids and is not qualified to practice medicine or to give prescriptive advice.

Readers should refer to a medical practitioner or qualified specialist clinician before acting on any of the advice or observations contained herein.

The purpose of this book is to brief readers on the research and to offer subject matter for further clinical research and thought leadership. As it stands, this work is not entirely conclusive or exhaustive.

The author takes no responsibility for any errors or omissions this document may contain. While amino acids and antioxidants are generally non-prescription, they should still be treated as prescriptive medicine and a qualified pharmacist or qualified medical doctor or dietician's advice should be taken before consumption.

Author: Mr Lee Friend
Friend Biotech
Unit 2
43 Carol Street
London NW10HT
Mob: +44 07778143766
lee@friendbiotech.com

ISBNs:
Paperback: 978 1 80227 474 5
Hardback: 978-1-80227-604-6
eBook : 978-1-80227-475-2

Contents

DEDICATION

I dedicate this book to amino health pioneers such as Dr R. I. Horowitz, Dr Luca Pangrazzi and Dr Alexey Polonikov, and to all the other clinicians and researchers listed in the reference section. A further dedication to HRH Prince Charles, The Prince of Wales, Without His Highness personal energetic promotion and support of Organic foods I doubt many of the UK population would have even heard of the term Organic food, let alone respected its importance. One ponders on how many countless lives the use of organic foods in our diets has improved, extended or indeed saved, including, possibly - my own !

INTRODUCTION

This book is written to be generally understood both by the layperson and the clinician, so it is not entirely professional as a clinical narrative. This book is motivated to provoke thought and lead to further research and clinical study.

Covid-19, as for many people, will probably have left the reader with many unanswered questions as they seek to protect themselves and their families.

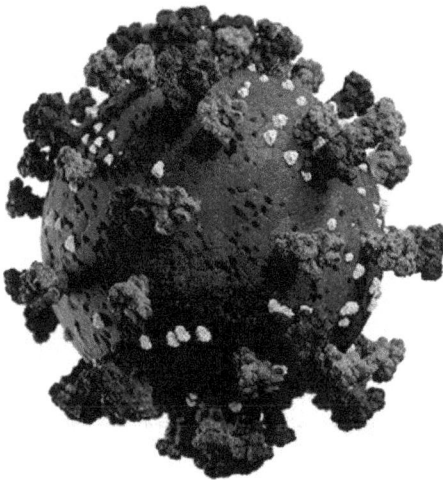

COVID-19

The questions

Why weren't you told that your immune system relies on proper nutrition as well as vaccines? Why was no guidance given?

Do you realise that the human body already has a natural defence to viruses including Covid-19, as evidenced by the majority of patients who recover quickly without needing any medical intervention? You can strengthen this defence system through diet and supplementation.

Do you know that your body has a built in self-destruct clock that automatically reduces the effectiveness of your immune system every year of your life? That is, unless *you* do something about it because it's unlikely that even your doctor will know about this.

Did you realise that alcohol—in the excessive consumption of alcoholic drinks—is one of the most toxic poisons you are likely to ingest? It can disable your immune system—just when you need it most—so why does no health warning about the risk of viral infections (as well as the risk of organ failure) come with it?

Could there have been a link between the First World War, the Spanish flu that killed millions and the extraordinary 13-year US prohibition on alcohol that followed?

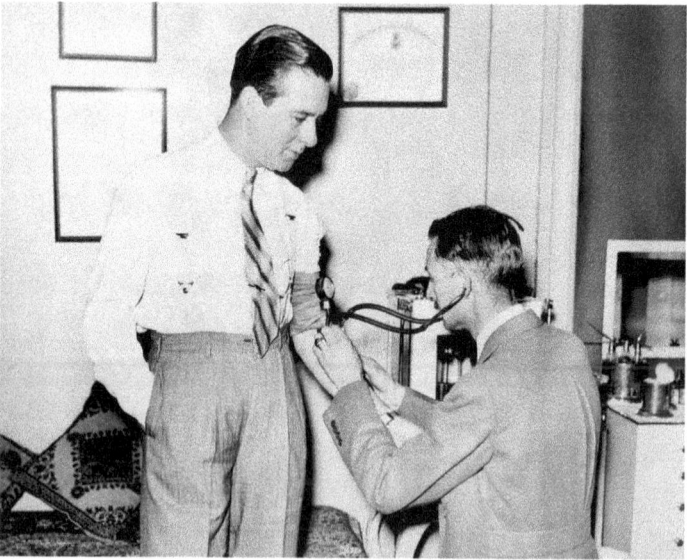

Did Donald Trump actually mean "Antioxidants" when referring to 'disinfectants' against Covid-19?

Are antibiotics being under-prescribed for the respiratory illness found in influenza patients? I'm sure many readers will have experienced the frustration of being refused antibiotics. Why does this happen?

The questions seem endless! Here are a few more, followed by some answers.

Why does an induced coma not always benefit recovery?

Why are the obese more vulnerable to Covid-19?

Why is diabetes a factor in Covid-19?

Why does this virus disproportionately affect the black community?

Why are younger, fitter people (aged 20–40) now being affected?

Why are all the stated Covid-19 high-risk groups more vulnerable?

Why? Why? Why?

Like many other academic medical researchers, I know the answers to these questions. Proven peer-reviewed research already exists and is backed by evidence mainly from existing respected academic clinical research; with much of it supported by *non-theoretical interventional* (actual human) *trials.*

Having discovered a common denominator in all Covid-19 high-risk or vulnerable groups, I've been able to identify potentially other unidentified high-risk groups. As the pre-existing conditions in these groups are possibly not yet recognised, they will be more susceptible to Covid-19.

The answers

Covid-19 can be a deadly predator which preys on the vulnerable and on groups at risk that are suffering from dietary deficiencies. Here, I will provide research evidence that suggests how the human immune system is quite capable of defeating this virus, as evidenced in the vast majority of people it infects who do not become critically ill.

In many cases, vaccines are vital in assisting the immune system and should be used except on qualified clinical advice to the contrary.

Even so, it is often assumed that vaccines are a cure-for-all, but a vaccine does not act as a mask or cloak that will keep a virus away. It will still enter the body. We rely on an efficient well-nourished immune system with its antioxidant levels normalised as this endogenous (produced by the body) defence will protect the body after the vaccine has performed its work; or to put it simply, after the body has 'recognised' the invader. If we gave a vaccine to a starving malnourished patient with other oxidative stress markers already swamping the immune system, our natural defences are far less likely to perform as intended, in conjunction with the vaccine.

The vulnerable groups need to be more aware of why they need to supplement their diet with non-prescriptive supplements to support their immune system—not only with vitamins—as these are only a part of the immune system's requirements, but also with minerals and amino acids. The importance of these appears to be largely forgotten.

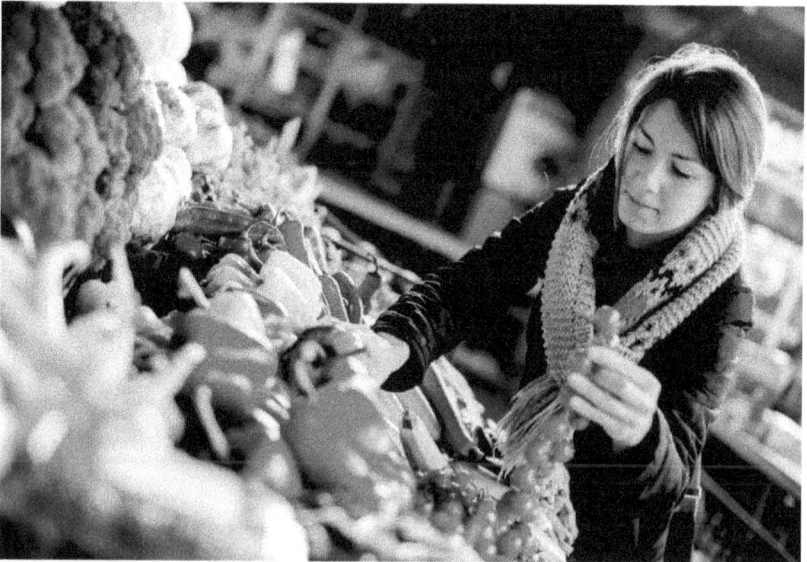

Part of the problem has been inevitable for a long time, the mission creep that was hidden in plain sight and has now clearly reached its critical mass or apex with the gradual breakdown of the immune system. We all knew that modern food processing, poor nutrition, factory farming and environmental toxicity would one day bite us, but not in the degenerative sense as cancer was viewed. Alzheimer's or coronary failure are not the direct results of a virus, but pneumonia lies latent within us all, and is ready to pounce when the immune system fails.

This situation is, in part, evidenced in the measurements of nutrition made around 1917 and again in 2017, where it was found that some fruit and vegetables that are generally available today, had, in certain instances, less than 70 percent of the nutritional value they had 100 years earlier.

In his ground-breaking book, *Nutrition and Physical Degeneration*, published as far back as 1939, Weston A. Price gave some grave early warnings of the consequences of placing profit before quality in food production. He observed the degradation and deterioration of the human body, accompanied by the over-reliance on medication. According to Price, the decline in health due to a poor diet from processed food and factory farming had already begun as far back as the early 1900s.

Although Price regularly refers to vitamins and minerals, I noted that he does not mention amino acids, which shows the recency of some of the research in Biochemistry. Nonetheless, I would invite the reader to read the clear warnings published in Price's book and his references to the poor diet that consisted of sugar, white flour, refined vegetable oils and processed canned foods. The lower immunity that resulted, then led to the sudden increase in infections from lung bacteria, such as tuberculosis and also dental decay.

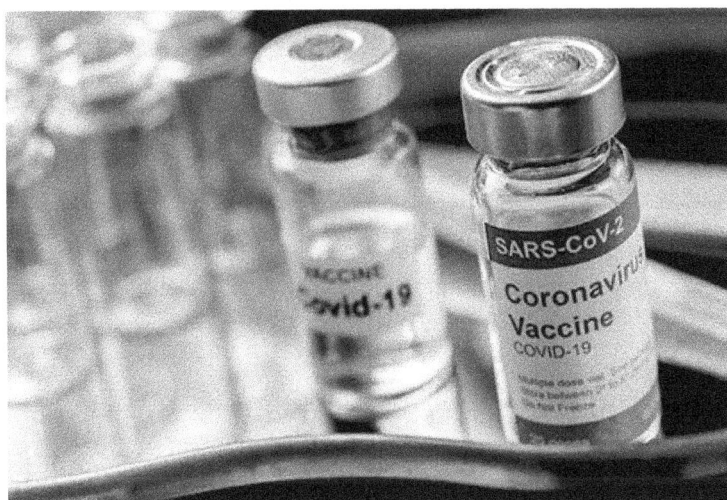

I would maintain today—some 83 years on from Weston Price's observations in 1939—that sugar, white flour and refined vegetable oils, on their own or hidden in processed food, are still our greatest enemy in terms of reducing our immunity to disease. What's more, the obesity that develops in the initially young slim body mass from eating such junk food becomes a self-fuelled habit with consequences that can be deadly. Obesity further exacerbates an ineffective immune system, causing greater oxidative stress from burning more energy in a larger body mass. The obese body burns even more energy and requires further antioxidants to counter the excess oxidisation - the by-products of producing and burning energy in a diet already deficient in antioxidants, again fuelling disease. It's no wonder that obese and chronically obese people are particularly vulnerable to Covid-19. I will explain *oxidative stress* and give more details about antioxidants and their importance a little later.

Please don't dismiss me as a crazy conspiracy theorist, I am a researcher who has been researching amino acids for over 20 years. A quick review of this book will show the clinical science involved, with examples of human-testing interventional trials, rather than mere ideology or theory. I own and run a multinational business, with 400 staff, and in my spare time I pursue private medical research, largely to promote health and longevity for my family and staff.

After submitting my studies to the leading UK government public health advisors, as well as writing to the Head of the NHS, I was asked to contribute to the work of the UK Government's Covid Therapeutics Task Force (CTAP) as a contributor on the subject of the antioxidant Glutathione (GSH). While closely observing the efficacy of vaccines to give relevance to my research before submission, I was just too late to submit my final work or give my warnings regarding the possible degraded efficiency of the vaccine in some cases, particularly with regard to alcohol consumption, especially in younger Covid-19 patients. The work of CTAP had come to an end just two months before the Omicron variant surfaced.

My personal view was, and still is, that a vaccine will rely on a properly functioning normalised immune system that is provided with sufficient nutrition, and—in order to tackle changing virus mutations in the first instance—the human body is not helped by being further compromised by an excessive intake of alcohol or other defective or dysfunctional diet or environmental toxicity.

From the time of beginning my research into amino acids 20 years ago, I had never been seriously ill with any illness until I contracted like many others Covid-19 long before it was even recognised in December 2019. Deciding I could not rely on what I felt was a flawed system that took little account of the natural immune system and the amino acids as well as vitamins and minerals the Human body requires through the diet.

1. MY COVID-19 INFECTION

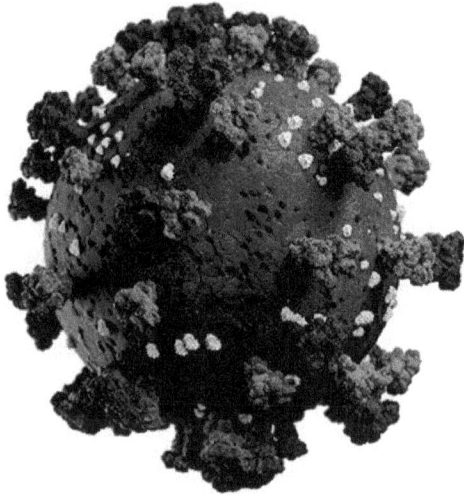

COVID-19

I realised, in December 2019, that the influenza outbreak now known as Covid-19, was more challenging than other flu viruses. Then, after a colleague returned from East Asia in the same month, I caught a throat and flu infection that made me slightly breathless and seriously fatigued. The whole office quickly caught what we all thought was a common winter bout of flu. I described it to my colleagues as a 'very dirty flu virus' and asked our international colleagues flying into the UK for Christmas not to attend work at the London office as it was so contagious.

As a relatively obese 62-year-old, and border-line diabetic, I take supplements and keep my RBC GSH (red blood cell glutathione) at around 2.8 mmol/l (average for my age 1.6 mmol/l). I increased my normal intake of amino acids and antioxidants and the virus symptoms disappeared within 3 days.

I appeared to have re-caught the infection during a skiing holiday in Austria 6 weeks later (probably from breakfast buffet tools which is a possible infection route for Covid-19 in hotels and cruise ships), collapsing while skiing due to a shortage of breath that I could not recover easily. I thought I'd either become unusually asthmatic or had a heart valve infection rather than having re caught the infection or suffered lung damage from just short exposure to Covid-19.the previous month.

I always carry dietary supplements as a common flu safeguard, and again, I self-treated with full-spectrum amino acids, full-spectrum vitamins, and with aminos based, glutathione and L-acetyl cysteine as antioxidants, as it was a respiratory infection. I bed rested and recovered in 2 days without assistance from doctors. A milder shortage of breath from the damage lasted for some time, which I treated with amino L-glutamine for long term muscle recovery.

I had no idea of the importance of this episode until Covid-19 was announced. As a researcher of aminos for over 20 years, I realised that my use of aminos had prevented escalation given my weight & age.

A blood test for IgG antibodies in May 2020 revealed that my staff and myself had no infected Covid-19 antibodies. I wasn't surprised—given that government guidance labs were testing for IgG type—when for a mild infection, an IgM response was more likely to be present.

Let me explain. An IgG (immunoglobulin G) is the most common antibody in the blood, an IgM is the first or primary antibody the body produces when it fights a new infection so is more likely to be present in mild cases that do not develop further; however that needs to be further confirmed by qualified clinicians.

2. A REMEDY IN PLAIN SIGHT?

It may well be that no serious blood testing and analysis of amino acid concentrations was ever undertaken in Covid-19 post-mortems, despite the clear evidential trail that points to the deficiency or depletion of particular master natural antioxidants (or 'disinfectants'). I understand routine post mortems were not permitted on COVID 19 victims in many countries. So for instance I do not know how clinicians determined the difference between the 70 000 terminally ill patients with smoking related diseases and their subsequent deaths that occur in the UK every year and COVID 19 as the cause of death, perhaps someone can enlighten me. Perhaps further because of the lack of post-mortems was this why it was not spotted that all the victims would have likely been seriously deficient in the bodies master antioxidant which I will go on to detail

This book is still a compromise. Short on deeper clinical details but with sufficient information to provide basic guidance to Clinical researchers, to clinicians, and in order to inform the layperson as simply as possible the importance of Amino nutrition using clinical research and cited evidence from interventional testing. It thereby provides subject matter for the readers' own research or even for desktop research in order to validate my claims.

Although a safeguard against the virus was and is at the time of writing hiding in plain sight, this cure may not provide sufficient financial incentives to large pharmaceutical companies unless Government support promotes greater awareness.

Importantly, from my research viewpoint, the Covid-19 virus does not randomly select its victims but specifically targets those with a weakness or with a depleted reserve of what is known as a 'tripeptide', a combination of three amino acids.

What's more, the virus not only affects the vulnerable elderly or people with pre-existing health conditions, but it is also affecting young persons with no so-called underlying conditions, but who may still be deemed as vulnerable. So why are the vulnerable, vulnerable? It's not just because they are old or obese —as many old and obese and vulnerable people survived—and why is it and was it, critically affecting only a minor percentage of the population?

Covid-19 is specifically targeting one particular weakness that is quietly hidden in plain sight.

My research indicated that there was only *one common denominator* among *all* the high-risk vulnerable groups, in *all* the critically or seriously affected, and in *all* the fatalities – the answer was:

Glutathione (GSH) deficiency

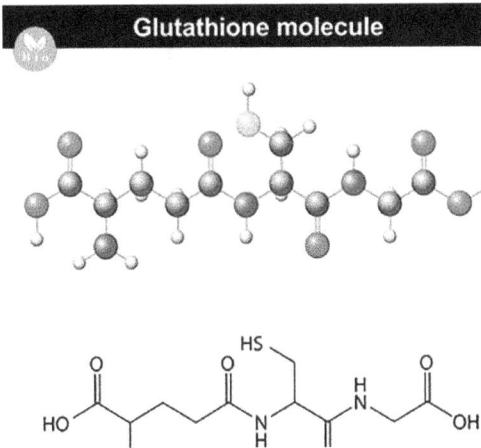

Glutathione molecule

GSH (glutamyl-cysteinyl-glycine) is the body's number one antioxidant (or 'disinfectant'). It is known as a tri-peptide due to its 3 amino-acid components:

- L-cysteine (CYS) (or NAC in N L acetyl form)

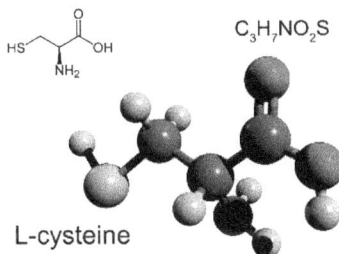

$C_3H_7NO_2S$

L-cysteine

- L-glycine (GLY)

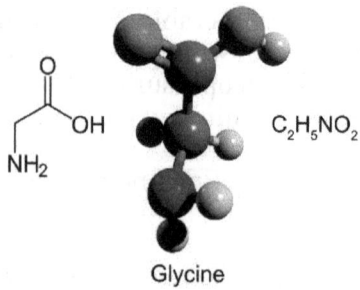

$C_2H_5NO_2$

Glycine

- L-glutamine (GLN)

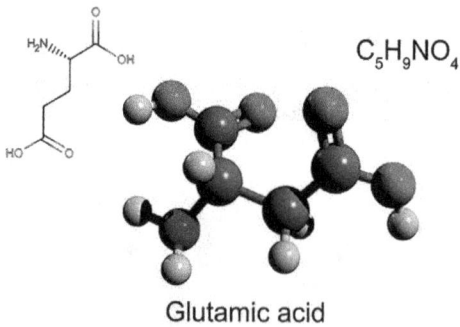

$C_5H_9NO_4$

Glutamic acid

Of the 3 components, CYS is the one most likely to be deficient and is, at the same time, the most important.

3. THE EVIDENCE: COVID-19 VULNERABLE GROUPS

Let us review all the vulnerable groups and their relationship to glutathione (GSH) and cysteine (CYS) deficiency. I will go into greater detail below on amino acids and antioxidants after presenting the evidence.

GSH and L-cysteine (CYS) deficiency is connected to *all* high-level Covid-19 risk groups, and potentially to risk groups still to be generally recognised, but which I have identified later in the book.

Covid-19 – diabetes & liver disease

The fact that around 26 percent of all COVID 19 fatalities are diabetic at the time of writing in 2020 should have rung alarm bells at the time !

GSH, which is stored in the liver, will not have sufficient synthesis or concentration in a damaged or impaired liver "Dysregulation of GSH synthesis is increasingly being recognized as contributing to the pathogenesis of many pathological conditions. These include diabetes mellitus, Pulmonary fibrosis, Cholestatic liver injury." [1]

Effects of age on glutathione depletion

GSH levels seriously decrease as the body ages. As we get older, we suffer from more oxidative stress, and this depletes the GSH needed to cope, making the elderly more susceptible to illness and disease without daily supplementation. In fact, after the age of 20, the availability of glutathione and other antioxidants naturally declines at an average rate of 10 percent per decade. Nonetheless, supplementation is rarely—if ever—applied.

Studies by Mitsubishi Life Sciences [2] demonstrate that the average decline in GSH RBC from the age of 20 is over 3.00 mmol/l. The level drops to the minimum WHO recommended level of 1.6 mmol/l by the age of 60. [2] Note: Mitsubishi Life Sciences produce a glutathione product under the brand name of Opitac.

At least one global multinational recognises the vital importance of GSH.

A second reason for the declining level of GSH is environmental pollution, such as the exhaust fumes and smoke we are exposed to daily. Further, the toxicity in processed foods such as sugar, vegetable oils and excessive alcohol use, all leads to a glutathione deficiency as Glutathione is used up in its dual role as a detoxifier. Additionally, the lack of nutritious homemade meals that include the recommended 7–9 servings of organic vegetables and fruit per day, when combined with the other factors, are all contributing factors.

Effects of glutathione depletion in obesity

Laboratory studies such as those of Sastre and Pallardo et al. [3] have proven that the condition of obesity lowers glutathione levels. At the same time, the higher levels of oxidative stress resulting from an excessive body mass also rapidly deplete the normal GSH reserves. Synthesis is further hindered by factors such as fatty liver stress issues, for instance (oxidative stress is simply the body's inability to control the balance or to regulate destructive cell oxidisation). Severely obese (BMI over 35) subjects have more extreme depletion of GSH, making them more susceptible to a whole range of health and immunity vulnerabilities such as Covid-19; hence the UK prime minister had a more extreme reaction than his slimmer colleagues. Given the vague press releases, I am assuming that not one doctor knew the actual reason, other than he was obese.

Whilst more research is needed, the evidence indicates that the amino-based immune system does not recognise or detect excessive body mass and does not synthesise extra antioxidants, including GSH, to cater for the higher-than-average mass ratio. Like the elderly, obese people need to supplement with amino acids daily, especially with the essential amino acids, in order to stay healthy.

Effects of glutathione depletion in black African Americans

Due to the genetic development among black African Americans, this group have lower glutathione levels than white people (the vulnerability of Asian or mixed ethnic groups needs further studies but is likely to be similar). Alana Morris A Morris MD, Liing Rijaz DDS Patel et al [4] noted "There was a trend toward more oxidized (depleted glutathione) in African Americans; however, this did not reach statistical significance After adjustment for demographics and CVD risk factors, [the] African-American race remained a significant correlate of lower glutathione levels."

Effects of glutathione deficiency on sense of smell

There are clear references to a connection between glutathione deficiency and olfactory dysfunction (impaired sense of smell). Researchers YH kim et al, have noted that induced GSH depletion in mice resulted in—again, induced and also age related GSH loss -resulted in the loss in the behavioural olfactory function. Ulrika Bergstrom et al, noted similarly inducing Glutathione depletion noted extensive damage to the Bowman Glands (olfactory Glands – our sense of smell glands [5] [6]

COPD effects of NAC (and GSH) levels on the 'cytokine storm' in the immune over-response typical in Covid-19 fatalities

Leading expert Dr Luca Pangrazzi at the University of Innsbruck noted that the "NAC [a component of GSH] can act as an antioxidant and anti-inflammatory drug by reducing cytokines and chemokines after influenza infection in [the] context of lower[ing] respiratory infection and targeting viral and bacterial infections." [7] Pangrazzi also reported that NAC and GSH regulate the response.

Furthermore, researchers at Baylor College of Medicine Houston, USA, found that N acetylcystiene helped combat Covid-19. They stated that NAC replenishes antioxidants to restore the normal response of immune cells, inhibiting T Cell apoptosis, and reducing the severity of pneumonia due to Covid-19 infection. [8]

Effects of glutathione deficiency on blood clotting

Blood-clotting issues were noted in seriously ill Covid-19 patients. Studies conducted in China by Dr Tong Qing Chen Et al noted the existence of "a direct and unquestionable linear relationship between blood-clotting function and levels of GSH which could be improved by glutathione supplementation in depleted subjects". [9]

4. COVID-19 VULNERABLE GROUPS NOT YET IDENTIFIED

It is my belief that there are more vulnerable Covid-19 groups yet to be discovered; vulnerable and risk groups whose immune system is further disabled and exacerbated by the following:

Glutathione synthetase deficiency

This is rare condition (around 70 patients worldwide) and disorder where the body is unable to synthesise glutathione. The symptoms are identical to Covid-19 – a shortage of breath and respiratory difficulties. This group is probably one of the most vulnerable, and sufferers would be unlikely to recover from a critical Covid-19 illness without a blood test to confirm zero vascular GSH and subsequent supplementation.

It would also suggest that all critical Covid-19 patients should have a GSH red blood cell test to ensure at least the minimum recommended RBC 1.6 mmol/l.

Helminth parasitic condition (worms)

Research in the US indicates that the majority of the population has some form of helminth parasites. So widespread is this condition that those free from it are usually only those who have already received treatment for such parasites. Further research indicates that, at times, up to 30 percent of the immune system is working to defend the body against parasitic worms, especially when dealing with the asymptomatic infections these parasites can cause.

Curiously, studies show that parasites use our GSH for their own protection, but further research is needed to prove that, in doing so, they can deplete our GSH. [10] In any case, however, any unnecessary load on an immune system tasked with Covid-19 needs to be tackled regardless.

Simple oral treatment using Mebendazole (trade names such as Vermox) is an anthelmintic anti worm medication used to remove and also treat infections caused by pinworm, roundworm, hookworm and whipworm, among other types.

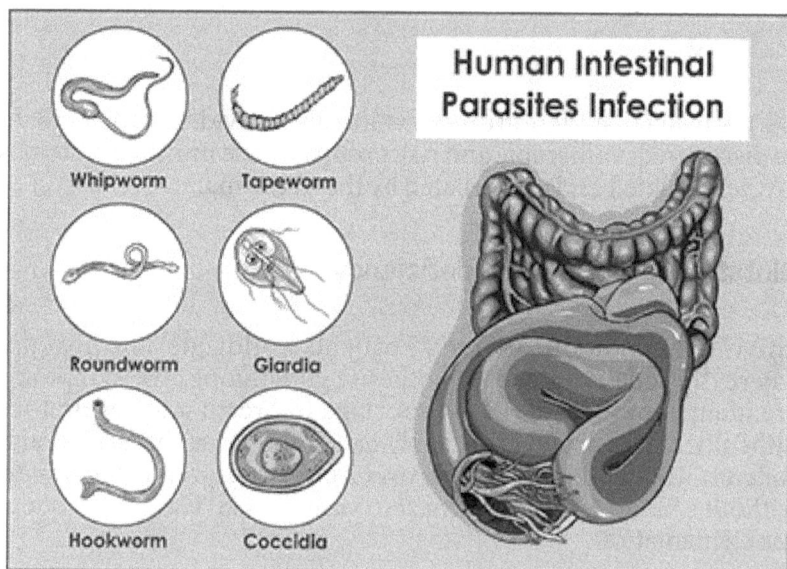

Whipworm

Tapeworm

Human Intestinal Parasites Infection

Roundworm

Giardia

Hookworm

Coccidia

Celiac or asymptomatic gluten-intolerant population

Gluten sensitivity goes largely unnoticed in the majority of those affected and is often asymptomatic. The symptoms possibly become more noticeable as a person ages or increases their gluten intake beyond their individual physiological capacity to cope; hence this might be a vulnerable group that is not very visible.

Celiacs are those with symptomatic gluten intolerance, and having identified the condition clinically, they will have largely reduced the problem by refraining from gluten. For this reason, this group may not appear in an identifiable Covid-19 spike, as addressing their gluten intolerance as a celiac they may have counteracted much of their vulnerability.

In his book, *Grain Brain,* leading US dietician and neurologist Dr David Perlmutter noted how multiple studies have proved that celiacs lose their ability to produce antioxidants, and have reduced levels of glutathione in particular, as a result of the immune system's response to gluten. [11]

Alcohol consumption, alcoholism and GSH

It may come as a surprise to many that. although its use is often taken for granted, alcohol—when taken in excess—is one of the most toxic substances a human can ingest. Following the intake of alcohol, the body immediately begins to convert the alcohol into acetaldehyde to protect itself. Simultaneously, the liver prioritises the detoxification process, essentially shutting down all other functions to deal with the toxicity, given that alcohol is potentially lethal, until the substance is removed through the digestive system. The immune system appears sufficiently intelligent to prioritise the biggest threat to the survival of the organism.

So, the alcoholic drink imbibed—whether in the form of a fashionable brand drink or otherwise—is actually a poison! The alcohol needs to be detoxified or metabolised urgently by an enzyme in the liver known as alcohol dehydrogenase (ADH). This enzyme breaks the alcohol down into acetaldehyde and then another enzyme breaks this down into the less harmful acetate for elimination from the body as quickly as possible.

A liver stressed by excessive alcohol ingestion will, simply put, reduce the ability of this organ to produce GSH and therefore to utilise all the reserves in the immune system. GSH, which is concentrated and synthesised in the liver, will be utilised to clear the toxicity, making the body vulnerable to infection by any virus or bacteria during, and following, the period of toxicity, until the levels of antioxidants such as GSH are re-established.

Subsequently, drinking alcoholic drinks in an infectious environment is possibly one of the worst scenarios for anyone. From a rational point of view, in fact, it is highly irresponsible—or even suicidal. The tendency to do so regardless may explain the Covid-19 spike in 22–44 year-olds after lockdown eased. It was this group that actually began the trail to discovering the gradual reduction in glutathione levels—and therefore in immunity due to aging (10% reduction every 10 years after age 20). At the same time, many people in this group also moved towards alcoholism during the first lockdown a habit and addiction that may well have continued long after.

The drastic increase in alcohol consumption during lockdown has now exposed a group that were not previously vulnerable, pre-lockdown, when their alcohol intake may have been more moderate. With the easing of lockdown, the surge in social activity, accompanied by even more exceptional drinking and new close contact with infected people in social environments, the higher rate of infection is not surprising. This is especially true as many sufferers may already have liver impairment or damage from such continuous exceptional alcohol usage. It was reported that alcoholism in the UK increased by 20 percent after the first lockdown.

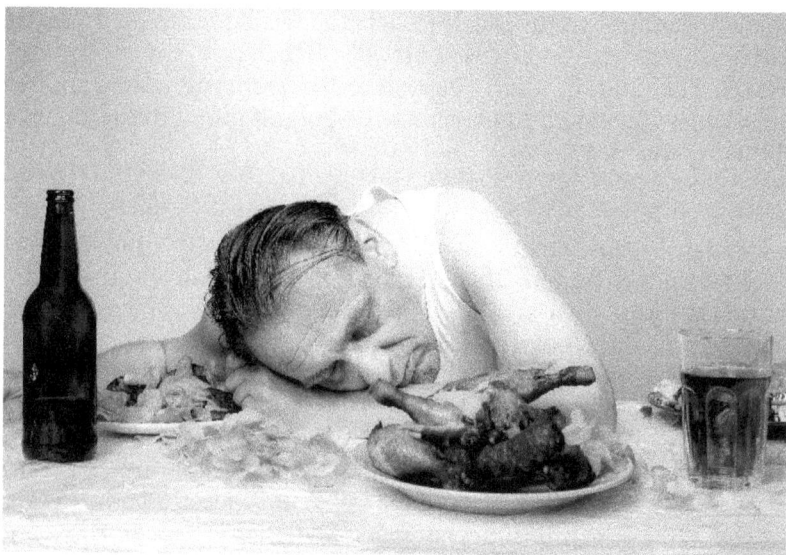

In their research on the relationship between GSH depletion and alcoholics and cirrhotic patients, Loguercio and Piscopo et al. reported: "Chronic alcohol abuse [as well as the subsequent], liver disease, induces a decrease of hepatic Glutathione (GSH). Treatment [supplementing with GSH] only made an improvement on those who abstained from alcohol [both during and after GSH supplemental treatment]." [12]

Let me pose a question. Why did the US introduce Prohibition in 1920 just as the Spanish flu pandemic ended? Lasting for 13 years,

Prohibition forbade citizens from selling, using or buying alcohol, despite the huge cost to the government in lost tax revenue. Could this perhaps be a tale, largely untold, of the discovery that a high alcohol intake had fuelled the spread of Spanish flu? I have no evidence to support this view, so perhaps it can make an interesting research subject for further investigation. Failing that, it could be used as part of a fictional film screenplay.

Patients with mercury amalgam dental toxicity

A relationship exists between the toxic haemoglobin (Hg) blood burden created by mercury amalgam dental fillings and L-cysteine – again let us not forget that L-cysteine is the most important and rarest precursor amino of GSH, and the most important single amino for respiratory illness defence.

It is likely that L-cysteine is being used and potentially depleted by the body's attempts at chelation (Chelation means to grab or bind and eliminate from the body) by using L-cysteine (whether nature's intention or not) to eliminate the mercury Hg toxicity by binding it to sulphur elements in the mercury blood toxicity so as to pass it out through the urinary system.

Studies, by the clinical scientists mentioned below, on patients' blood mercury levels confirm that with NAC (N L-acetyl cysteine) and selenium supplementation, it is possible to largely reduce the mercury Hg blood toxicity.

Without supplementation, it is clear that the body's normal reserves will bind to sulphur elements and deplete the ordinary levels of L-cysteine available to the immune system and for GSH synthesis, potentially causing a breakdown in the immune system defence structure. Clinical studies by Hibberd, Howard et al. and Spiller et al. confirm this position. [13, 14]

It would be useful to look at the percentage of Covid-19 fatalities to see if there is a correlation between with mercury or plastic filings.

It might also be useful to look at the percentage of Japan's population with mercury fillings, for example, or at other countries where better recovery rates have been seen. Conversely, identifying this percentage in poorer nations with unusually high critical infection rates could also be useful.

At the same time, the removal of mercury fillings would not be advisable in critical patients without exceptional care to prevent the huge toxic spike potentially caused by extraction. This danger should be considered in all vulnerable groups, including the obese.

Again, in isolation, the toxicity in mercury fillings may not be very significant, but when combined with any of the other vulnerability factors mentioned, however, it could contribute to critical illness and to the worst outcomes of Covid-19.

CLA (conjugated Linoleic Acid Deficiency)

Further factors affecting GSH synthesis include dis-regulation caused by diet, genetics or C19 virus activity, as well as linoleic acid (LA) and conjugated linoleic acid (CLA) deficiency.

Researchers at the German Cancer Research Centre, Heidelberg proved that LA, an omega fatty acid in conjugated form (CLA), can up-regulate or increase the synthesis of GSH. Their study concluded that: "Conjugated Linoleic Acid unlike other unsaturated fatty acids strongly induces Glutathione synthesis without lipo peroxidation." [15]

A conjugated linoleic acid (CLA) is produced by ruminant bacteria as an intermediate of the polyunsaturated fatty acids of linoleic acids.

In simple terms, lipid peroxidation is a process in which a radical abstracts an electron from an unsaturated fatty acid to create an unstable lipid radical that can cause serious damage to cell membranes. CLA enhances and up-regulates GSH synthesis without any adverse reaction.

The existing studies from the German Cancer Research Centre may provide a shortcut for research into how and to what extent that CLA regulates GSH, so that further research can focus on why and how the C19 virus may benefit from such a molecule, which may be indicative of a man-made virus.

Effect of induced coma on glutathione and the immune system

The drugs typically used to clinically induce coma are Propofol, barbituates and opioids.

Propofol does not affect GSH synthesis, as indicated by clinical research for this drug. It is used as a primary induction agent and may not be administered continuously for the long-term maintenance of the patient's coma state.

Barbiturates are regarded by the body as toxic, as shown in research. These drugs affect GSH regulation and synthesis as the GSH synthesised is used and prioritised to detoxify. Without the supplementation of GSH, barbiturates could harm the effectiveness of GSH to promote an adequate immune system response.

Opioids have also been shown in research to be regarded by the body as toxic, and affect GSH regulation and synthesis as, again, the GSH already synthesised in the body is used and prioritised to detoxify. Unless GSH is supplemented, these drugs could therefore undermine the effectiveness of GSH, resulting in an inadequate immune system response.

For the layman, an induced coma is not achieved by a single dosing but is continuously dosed to maintain the coma condition. The immune system will attempt to detoxify and eliminate the toxic substances using GSH.

Note that this observation is not meant as a criticism of any critical care prescription of induced coma. Indeed, where other factors such as patient comfort and the urgent emergency uplifting of blood oxygen levels are concerned, these considerations may override the requirement for GSH and the immune system to fight the virus at that point. Long-term use may, however, may be counter-productive to recovery and may contribute to long-term ICU occupancy and high mortality rates.

It is unknown if supplementation of GSH or its precursors was completely part of the prescriptive care plan in the IV nutrition support. It may be counter-productive to assist the body to eliminate barbiturates and opioids by natural GSH detoxification, as this may reduce the effect of the drug itself and may require the need for a higher dosing, thereby creating a deadly cycle. (This would require confirmation by a qualified Biochemist)

Furthermore, the observation regarding the use of continuous positive airway pressure apparatus (CPAP) (a machine used for patients who stop breathing while in deep sleep) without an induced coma may allow a better performance from the immune system for recovery needs qualified peer reviews. Indeed, as clinicians have become more experienced with Covid-19 treatment, it has been reported that induced coma is no longer the first choice of treatment and, in order to assist breathing, CPAP machines with O2 supplementation, which did not require drugs to induce coma were preferred to induced coma.

Black fungus

As the latest Covid-19 *hot potato,* the outbreak of 'black fungus' (mucormycosis) in India may be indicative of an immune system—already burdened with oxidative stress—dealing with diabetes and Covid, again creating a huge challenge, as noted by Camara-Lemarroy et al. [16] These patients also have decreased phagocytic activity due to an impaired glutathione pathway. The blood acidosis condition (when the blood is too acidic) that accompanies black fungus leads the kidneys to 'rob' the immune system of vital nutrients, especially glutathione. By reducing the availability of GSH in the immune pathway, the effect of Covid-19 could be deadly.

5. EVIDENCE SUMMARY - VULNERABLE GROUPS

By the time a patient is seriously ill with Covid-19—given the body's initial attempt to defend itself—GSH levels would already be depleted. Having commenced the fight with already reduced GSH capacity and potentially deficient amino-rich nutrition in food, it becomes a one-sided battle. When the GSH tri -peptide precursor components of NAC, GLU, GLY aminos are depleted and become 'conditional', the body will begin 'scavenging' from food ingestion. If it finds the 'larder bare' of the nutritional conditional aminos required for synthesis the body will be unable to defend itself properly using GSH

If, therefore, a diagnosis of Covid-19 was made on a super-computer set to pure logic (rather than to "commercial or vaccine solutions only"), the computer could be expected to spot the common denominator immediately. Clearly, such logic is not currently being applied.

At the same time, the industry is looking in the direction of an expensive 'catch all' vaccine that may fail if the virus mutates too widely. Also, without supplementation of the GSH component to assist the immune system with new challenges, this vaccine may also fail. The immune system is akin to a super-computer capable of adapting its own defences to mutations. We can deduce this fact because the immune system has saved us from extinction without medical assistance for thousands of years as far as the amino-immune structure is intact.

Let us not forget that the 1918 Spanish flu did not just simply disappear. With no assistance from antibiotics or antiviral drugs, as these were yet to be invented, it is likely that once the very vulnerable groups had largely either died or recovered, our immune system actually defeated the virus for the vast majority of the remaining world population. The Spanish flu, incidentally, is now known to have been a variant of H5N1 'bird flu'.

The action of GSH and its components NAC, glutamine and glycine, which would have been in the front line of the defence against Spanish flu, may explain why the human race had some form of resistance to the recent H5N1 infection. As a respiratory infection, this did not turn into a pandemic as it could have done like Covid-19, because nothing has changed in aminos and antioxidants in the 100 years since the Spanish flu and their action and importance to aid the immune system. We therefore need to be more confident in the amino immune system as it probably saved the human race from extinction then.

Covid-19 Vulnerability GSH Checklist *See Appendix*

Vaccines

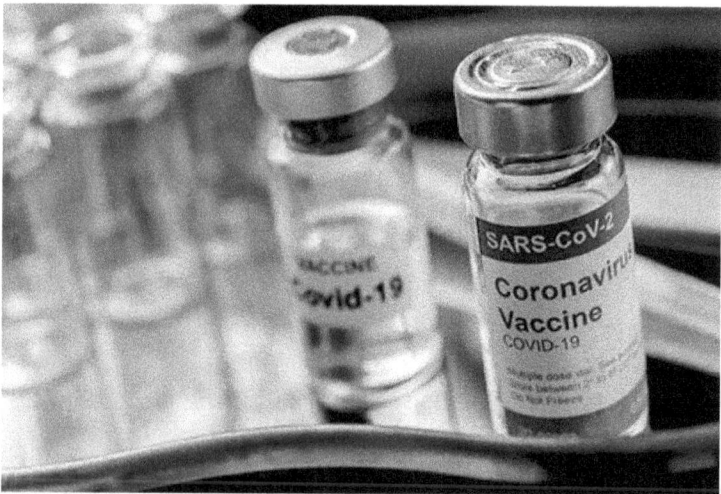

No current document or book on Covid-19 would be complete without some reference to vaccines, which at the time of writing are produced using in two types of technology. One, from Astra Zeneca, is based on the traditional flu-type inactive virus cell injection that triggers the immune system to attack similar virus cells. The other, from Pfizer and Moderna, among other companies, is the mRNA (messenger RNA).

Used in cancer treatments since 2011, mRNA instructs the body into making the Corona virus spike protein, which triggers an immune system response. There are some public concerns that if, during its implementation, this technology attacked or risked attacking other similar but helpful corona-type viruses existing happily in the human body (known as retro-viruses) that are vital for instance to the health of the female reproductive system.

For example, Syncytin which as a Corona virus itself enables a foetus to be carried internally within the human by protecting it from other virus and bacteria and is a difference between the human body and Reptilians for instance who without Syncytin to assist do not carry foetus internally and lay eggs. Of course this factor or risk would be well known to the pharmaceutical companies and their Bioscientists would, subsequently, have conducted a large scale risk assessment of the short term and long-term effects of such biotechnology.

The manufacturers and their scientists have been quoted as saying the mRNA is very specific, as it targets very specific corona virus spike proteins, not *all* corona viruses, There have been no reported cases whatsoever of any such detriment during the vast year long multinational vaccine use. Given spike proteins are made of aminos I noted one journalist say given there are only 20 aminos how can this be safely targeted? This view is incorrect, the Standard 20 (or 22) proteinogenic aminos referred to are a small fraction of all known aminos and combinations of aminos (peptides) which would likely have been utilised to get a spike protein DNA match, I refer to proteinogenic aminos in later chapters.

While concerns are often based on fears of runaway responses the actual weakness reported with mRNA is conversely in what is referred to its "Short tail "IE its very limited and short life. mRNA activity can be further regulated and controlled by the use of Micro RNA, mRNA, as potential safeguard which is relatively new science, so I have very little knowledge of same

Quick bioscience lesson for those that are still understandably confused! The principle simple difference then between traditional Astra Zeneca type vaccine is it produces inert inactive or dead virus cells" In Vitro" (in a glass jar) in a laboratory which are then injected into the human body the mRNA based vaccines are based on producing sending an instruction to the body via an injected DNA message to produce inert inactive or dead virus cells "Endogenously" (within the human body)

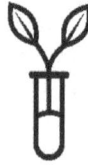

BIOTECHNOLOGY

The Immune System Response

Simply put the immune system works in part by utilising what are known as *macrophages*. These are large, vital specialist cells of the immune system—formed in response to an infection—that recognise (thanks in part to the help of vaccines), engulf and retard the multiplication of neighbouring virus cells by destroying the infected virus cells using *interferons*, the proteins that actually inhibit the replication of virus cells. Macrophages and the complete immune system structure response involving T Cell and other mechanisms would be the topic of an entire book and given that the focus of this book is on nutrition and glutathione, I will not go into depth other than to show the further relevance of GSH to macrophages by quoting from recent scientific research by Marina Diotallevi Paola Checconi et al at the Brighton and Sussex Medical School Brighton, UK. "Glutathione fine tunes the innate Immune system response towards antiviral pathways in MacroPhage cells – independently of its antioxidant properties."

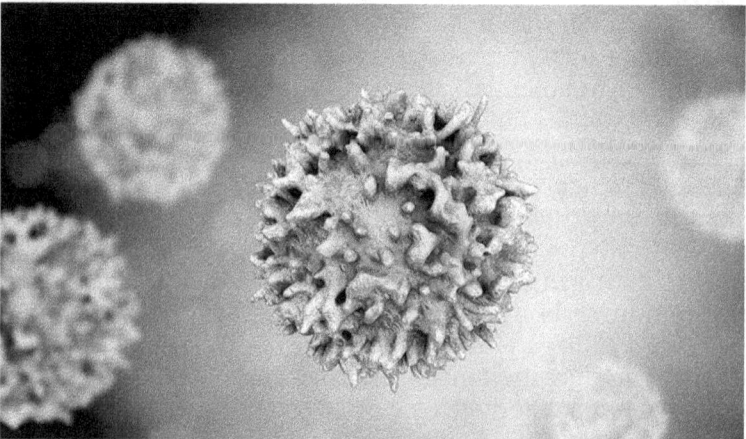

There follows an explanation of the 'independent antioxidant properties' referred to by some of the researchers quoted above. When the immune system rallies to fight intruders, the oxygen it uses produces a massive volume of free radicals that, for a change, may become helpful in destroying viruses and bacteria in an oxidative oxidised cell explosion. Without sufficient antioxidants such as glutathione to absorb excess free radicals, however, this event may become unregulated, harming the body and its immune system response. Again we see the importance of GSH to an immune system that is fit-for-purpose with fine-tuned responses.

You may already have heard of *cytokine storms*. Cytokines are small immune system messenger cells that may, in certain conditions—in an uncontrolled free radical situation perhaps (needs confirming research)—cause too strong a response from the immune system. This can result in the blood vessel walls opening up to let in immune cells such as interferons, which causes fluid to fill the lungs, harming the patient, often fatally. Research by Dr Luca Pangrazzi shows that cysteine, a component if glutathione, also helps to regulate the cytokine response. [7]

6. GSH AND ITS COMPONENT AMINO ACIDS

Discovered in 1888, Glutathione is a critical antioxidant found in all *eukaryotic* cells (cells that have a nucleus enclosed in a membrane, as found in humans and plants, for example. (Technically glutathione is known in chemistry as a type of *thiol,* which is an organic compound containing a sulphur analogue of an alcohol, hence the SH). Higher GSH concentrations protect against cellular damage, tissue degeneration, and disease progression in various models. In layman's terms, GSH is an antioxidant that inhibits free radical or discarded electrons and other toxins from energy production and use that would, if left unchecked, cause oxidation damage to other cells.

Jackson AA, Gibson NR, Lu Y, Jahoor [28] noted in their research, "Many pathological conditions are associated with decreased GSH levels This could be due to several reasons. For instance, oxidative stress could cause GSH loss though oxidation. **Another important aspect is nutrition**, as it was shown that, even when dietary protein intake is sufficient for maintaining nitrogen balance, it may not be sufficient for maintaining cellular GSH, particularly in conditions of oxidative stress. "

We will deal with the term "Oxidative stress" further on

GSH is not currently sold with any real vigour (apart from in Japan and some other parts of Asia), as an oral supplement. As mentioned, GSH is a tri-peptide, which means it is made up of three component amino acids. Oral supplementation of its individual components, such as L-glutamine, is *not* the most efficient option due to its degradation in the stomach when ingested. Together, the three component amino acids L-acetyl cysteine (NAC), glycine (GLY) and L-glutamine (GLN) are more digestively robust and enhance GSH synthesis, making GSH better absorbed and therefore more suitable for oral supplementation if the 3 component amino acids are taken individually. Liposomal GSH is an effective form for oral supplementation. It is encapsulated in a sheath of fats with lecithin and other elements to help it survive the acidity as it passes through the stomach to be absorbed in the intestine.

NAC on its own is known to assist in reducing fatalities in respiratory disease and glutamine is used by athletes for muscle repair. Both should be used to recuperate lung-damaged patients: NAC will assist in the emphysema phase, and glutamine—preferably L-acetyl glutamine—will assist in the later stage repair of lung fibrosis damage.

It is highly likely that the GSH tri-peptide and its three component amino acids would be depleted in all Covid-19 fatality post-mortems. The combination of this tri-peptide of 3 amino acids (or precursors) synthesises the body's master antioxidant glutathione. These names are not new to the medical profession and knowledgeable researchers will note the same factors present as in the immune system pandemic HIV Aids, where the virus was acted to prevent glutathione absorption through the cell barriers.

When the body is undergoing an illness crisis, glutathione is required in far greater volume than can ordinarily be created by the body itself or through its food resources, which are largely depleted of nutrients already in the fast food and supermarket food today, hence perhaps a valid explanation for the escalation in Covid-19 illness.

Brief explanation of aminos for the layman

Our body requires around 20 Standard aminos, referred to as "Proteinogenic" aminos. The word Proteinogenic means "Protein Creating" in all known life there are 20 genetically encoded (proteinogenic) amino acids and an additional further 2 that can be incorporated via conversion processes. Proteinogenic aminos are only a small fraction of all known aminos and combinations known as peptides. These standard aminos in simple terms make up the protein that you eat, or your body synthesises, and your body tissue is made of.

Let us note that we can survive without Carbohydrate but not without protein and fats. Protein is the only macronutrient to contain nitrogen without same we cannot grow or reproduce and the recommended protein input per day is 0.8 g per kilogram of body weight. If you strip away water and fat, protein makes up the majority of your body weight. There are 9 Standard Proteinogenic aminos that are the building blocks of human tissue

About half of the 20 standard amino s are termed *essential* or *indispensable* and the other half termed *dispensable* or *non-essential* and some which are further regarded as *Conditional*

'Complete aminos' often refers wrongly to complete essential aminos as it is often felt that one can ignore the non-essential aminos as the body will make them. A full-spectrum amino-acid supplement or preparation means a combination of all 20 standard essential and non-essential aminos.

Essential amino acids: obtained from food intake

Dispensable or non-essential amino acids: synthesised by the body

Conditional amino acids: are non-essential aminos that have to be obtained from food when the body is unable to synthesise the volume required when, for instance, the body is under stress with acute or chronic illness. These include the cysteine, glutamine, glycine and GSH tri-peptide components; hence the importance of diet or amino supplementation for the immune system to function effectively.

20 amino acids
A life basis

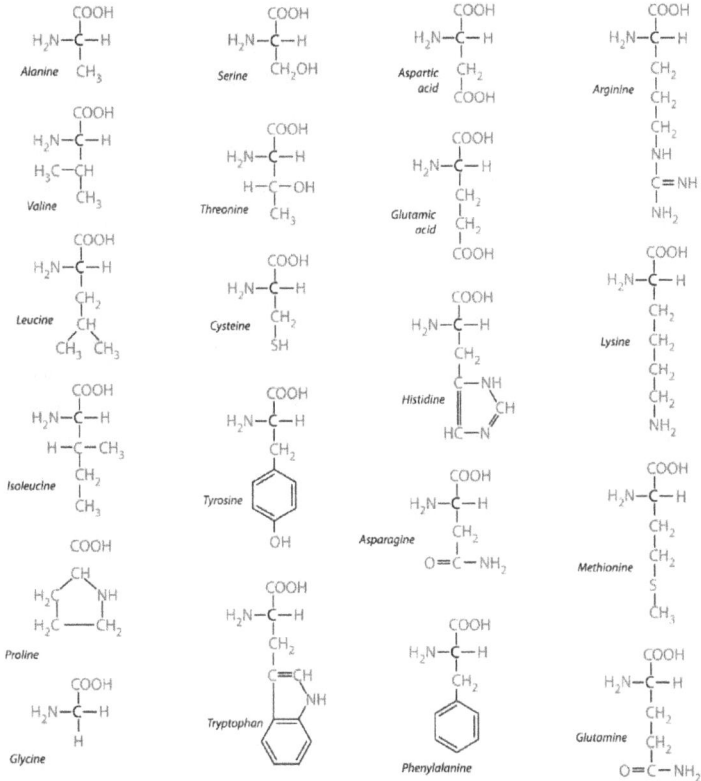

Alanine — H$_2$N—C—H, COOH, CH$_3$

Valine — H$_2$N—C—H, H$_3$C—CH, CH$_3$, COOH

Leucine — H$_2$N—C—H, CH$_2$, CH, CH$_3$ CH$_3$, COOH

Isoleucine — H$_2$N—C—H, H—C—CH$_3$, CH$_2$, CH$_3$, COOH

Proline — COOH, CH, H$_2$C, NH, H$_2$C—CH$_2$

Glycine — H$_2$N—C—H, H, COOH

Serine — H$_2$N—C—H, CH$_2$OH, COOH

Threonine — H$_2$N—C—H, H—C—OH, CH$_3$, COOH

Cysteine — H$_2$N—C—H, CH$_2$, SH, COOH

Tyrosine — H$_2$N—C—H, CH$_2$, OH, COOH

Tryptophan — H$_2$N—C—H, CH$_2$, C=CH, NH, COOH

Aspartic acid — H$_2$N—C—H, CH$_2$, COOH, COOH

Glutamic acid — H$_2$N—C—H, CH$_2$, CH$_2$, COOH, COOH

Histidine — H$_2$N—C—H, CH$_2$, C—NH, HC—N, CH, COOH

Asparagine — H$_2$N—C—H, CH$_2$, O=C—NH$_2$, COOH

Phenylalanine — H$_2$N—C—H, CH$_2$, COOH

Arginine — H$_2$N—C—H, CH$_2$, CH$_2$, CH$_2$, NH, C=NH, NH$_2$, COOH

Lysine — H$_2$N—C—H, CH$_2$, CH$_2$, CH$_2$, CH$_2$, NH$_2$, COOH

Methionine — H$_2$N—C—H, CH$_2$, CH$_2$, S, CH$_3$, COOH

Glutamine — H$_2$N—C—H, CH$_2$, CH$_2$, O=C—NH$_2$, COOH

Attitudes towards amino acid supplementation

As there is no space here to give a detailed explanation of all 20 standard amino acids, I have focused on the three amino components of GSH as some of the most important for the immune system.

Let's be honest and admit that 'vitamin' is a much more marketable name for a supplement than 'amino acid'! Essentially, much of the world fails to supplement with GSH, which is actually one of our body's protein building blocks that enables it to function both physically and mentally, and is vital to the body's own built-in defence – the immune system.

Let us again remind ourselves that our immune system has kept our species alive for thousands of years without any medical assistance, and our race has not been wiped out or erased from the Earth by any virus or bacteria to date.

Antibiotics only appeared in the 1930s, after our immune system had defeated the Spanish flu pandemic – and yet here we are in 2022, hiding out in our homes waiting for a vaccine or an antibiotic for a flu virus when we have an immune system like a super-computer. If fed properly to maintain its structure, the immune system can tackle the Covid-19 minor flu illness in the vast majority of the global population. As we are well aware not all the unvaccinated that caught the infection required hospitalisation or died proving a fit immune system can work, however without GSH Testing freely available or an immune system assessment being utilised many unvaccinated were without knowing vulnerable and died so currently some form of vaccination is necessary, the future should be based on immune system assessments and better knowledge of what makes the vulnerable groups vulnerable.

7. PURPOSE OF GSH AND VITAMINS IN THE IMMUNE SYSTEM

Vitamins support glutathione and other antioxidants in supporting the immune system. Vitamin E, for example, acts in a similar way to vitamin C – it recycles glutathione and depends on it for proper functioning and recycling as well as Selenium, Vitamins B6, B12, B1 and B2 are also required in the synthesis and recycling of GSH. B1 and B2 maintain GSH and its related enzymes in their active forms.

The latest study, published in 2013 with 54 healthy adults, registered for the first time a 30–35 percent increase in GSH levels only after 6 months of supplementing with basic oral glutathione at 1000mg per day – so basic oral GSH combination is *not* the best means of GSH treatment. It does not survive the digestive journey well and takes time to build up within the body.

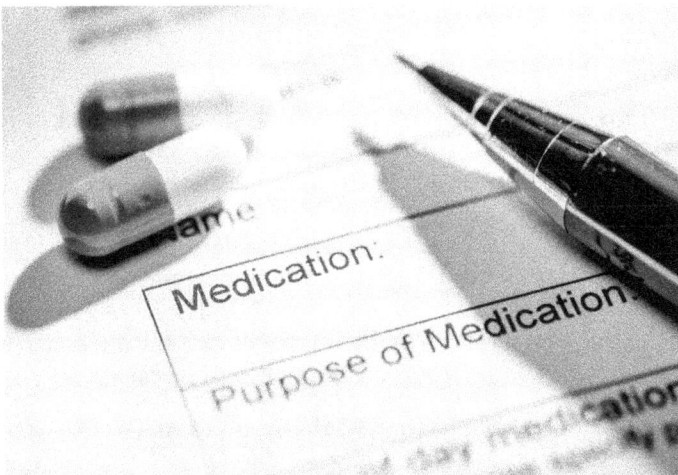

8. IMMUNE SYSTEM MANAGEMENT

Covid-19 relies on a weak immune system and a lack of understanding of the real importance of amino acids in health, starting at the GP education level. It seems that the average GP has received less than a couple of days education on a subject that is vital to our physical and mental health. All too often, the medical profession needs a marketable pharmaceutical cure or treatment for doctors to refer to.

At the same time, the immune system has it limits. Its loading has to be managed and reduced or assisted at certain times. Working largely unnoticed, it defends the body against an armada of infections, pathogens, viruses, and bacteria. We only notice the actions of our immune system when it becomes overloaded and takes noticeable action such as raising the temperature in an effort to impede the efficacy of the invader and to prompt fatigue in order to ensure we preserve energy and reduce oxidative stress.

Antibiotics

It is curious how Doctors are reluctant to prescribe antibiotics for influenza, stating that it is effective only in bacterial infections and not viruses, The result is the risk of the flu developing into bronchitis and pneumonia and indeed viral Pneumonia given the most common cause of such is - the Flu, a condition given the high transmissibility of COVID 19 and a seriously weakened immune system was a simple step through for COVID 19. As many of us know, the flu condition normally improves quickly after a course of antibiotics. Let us look at some evidence-based research.

A study led by Dr Marc Miravitlees [17] noted that:

- 18 percent of clear sputum tested positive for bacterial infection

- 59 percent of green sputum tested positive for bacterial infection
- 46 percent of yellow sputum tested positive for bacterial infection

How many patients are offered a lab analysis of their sputum? Without a test, the majority of green sputum patients—probably the majority of patients attending GPs and presenting flu symptoms—may consequently have been misdiagnosed if not given antibiotics.

Perhaps we can also ponder on the cost of every flu patient being offered lab testing of their sputum to validate an antibiotic prescription, while keeping in mind the Latin phrase and legal term *cui bono* – who benefits? Who in fact benefits from patients being refused antibiotics or from not being offered a lab test of their sputum to validate the prescription? Certainly not the patient, whose general health and Covid-19 vulnerability may be at risk in such circumstances.

It may also be that antibiotics deal with other hidden asymptomatic bacterial infections and free the immune system to work on the wider bacterial and virus problems using its own antioxidants which are thereby in a more abundant supply.

We are told that issuing even basic broad-spectrum antibiotics such as Tetracycline risks resistance to recent powerful antibiotics. Given these first-generation antibiotics were introduced in the late 1950s. It was some 40 years later in the 1980s before the second generation, Ciproflaxin, for instance, was produced in order to bridge any resistance in some patients to the first-generation antibiotics. Given that antibiotics are there to save lives, how many people die every year from not being offered antibiotics at the influenza stage, as opposed to those that die of antibiotic resistance?

How many Covid-19 patients may have benefited from antibiotic treatments following an early diagnosis before they developed bronchitis and pneumonia? Certainly, a detailed study of this situation needs to be instigated and the assumption that giving antibiotics risks greater population fatalities via antibiotic resistance needs to be quantified by evidence-based peer-reviewed clinical studies. After all there is huge recent update to any previous research and data - given the millions that have died of COVID 19 and further given the COVID 19 started in the winter flu season and flu could have been the precursor with millions weakened by unresolved Flu or Bronchial conditions.

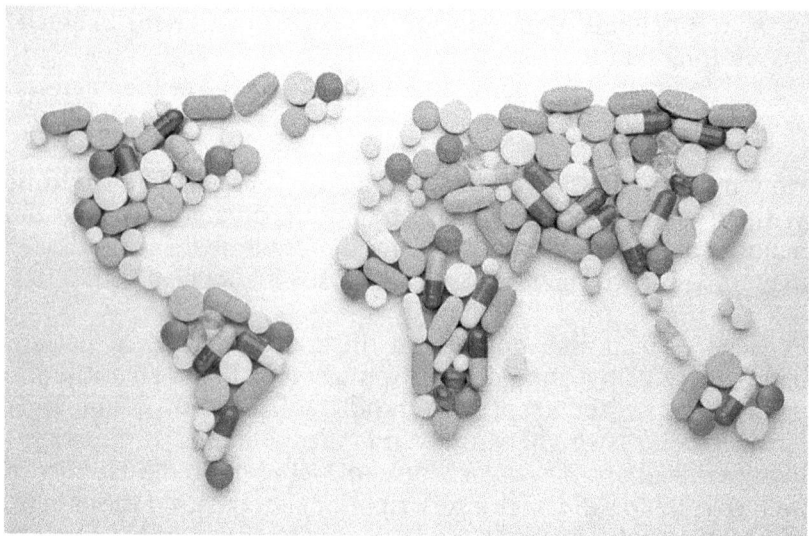

I will let the reader ponder this suggestion that could actually be viewed as frivolous by some government-backed academics. However, to return to our main subject, researchers at the Medical School, Sydney, Australia, noted that glutathione can, in certain instances, enhance antibiotic activity, but this detail is beyond the scope of this book. [18]

In terms of management, humans can do one thing to assist this powerful super-computer of a system – that is essentially to plug it into the mains supply by feeding it properly with amino acids as well as vitamins.

9. DESCRIPTION OF GLUTATHIONE FOR LAYPERSONS

Glutathione (GSH) is a critical endogenous (produced by the body) antioxidant used in protecting the body. It is found in all eukaryotic cells (cells where the nucleus is enclosed by a membrane) in humans, mammals and plants. Like a Swiss army knife, GSH has several important functions.

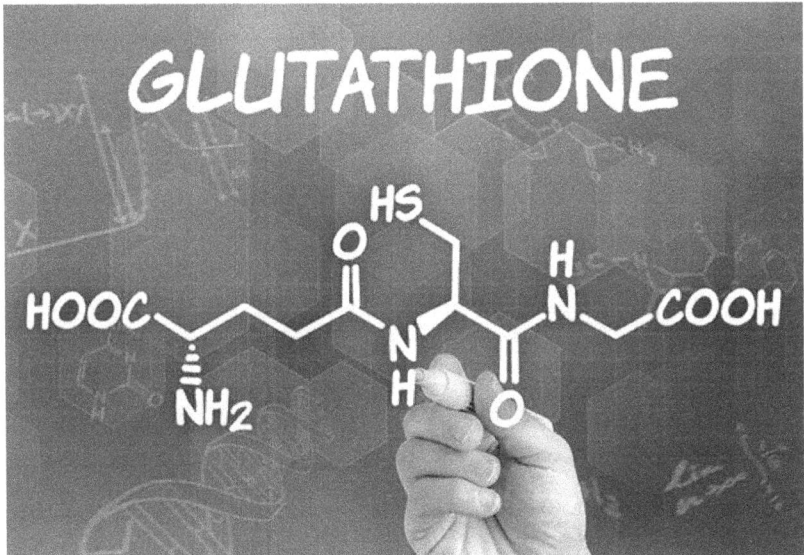

Higher GSH concentrations protect against cellular damage, tissue degeneration and disease progression as well as eliminating the toxicity in the body from alcohol, for example.

As an antioxidant, GSH neutralises the harmful electrons, known as free radicals, and other toxins created in energy production in cells, before they cause further damage by attaching to other cells.

Oxidative stress refers to the situation that occurs when antioxidants—usually by deficiency and signalling—fail to properly regulate the oxidisation of cells (*redox homeostasis*), which can result in cell death and disease.

Humans burn oxygen in *reactive oxygen species* (ROS) process in *Mitochondria* (energy cells) and in the same way as a fire blackens wood by oxidising it completely into carbon and carbon dioxide gas. This process prevents the by-products from overwhelming the wood fire, in which case it would no longer burn and would pollute and reduce the energy produced by the fire. The carbon (or ash) is carried away to ensure further combustion (perhaps an over simplified illustration). Essentially, we can look at GSH as chimney and filter working with other elements and substances to essentially clean, recycle and eliminate the bi products of energy production

Hence there is considerable interest within academic circles to develop interventions that augment GSH biosynthesis. Since the advent of Covid-19, however, it seems that the commercial resources are being diverted to vaccine solutions.

10. HEALTHCARE INDUSTRY

Covid-19, so what went wrong or did anything go wrong? How and why has the amino and GSH defence been missed by many national health organisations worldwide? Due to their limited education on this subject, GPs, as mentioned above, are largely ignorant of the detailed amino-acid functions and the effects of deficiencies.

Most medical researchers researching into GSH appear to be in university labs and are therefore more driven by academic study and theses than by commercial interests, perhaps. Many note that more investment is needed to properly research GSH and other antioxidants. Such investment is unlikely to come from pharmaceutical companies, however, as they will not be able to license or sell the result effectively without a demand for mass production.

Currently, there may be no real money for the pharmaceutical industry in this solution. As a common amino tri-peptide, GSH either cannot be licensed or a demand in population-sized volumes is first required. With government support, however, the pharmaceutical industry could profit from the mass production of aminos and antioxidants such as glutathione once there is volume appeal, in the same way as they profit from vitamins such as GSK and its Berrocca brand. The support from government would be in providing education and awareness to the public through advertising.

If the reader briefs an independent university professor of clinical researcher on the view presented here, it is unlikely to be disputed. It will be impossible to dispute the evidence given here or the recommendations made, whether by running basic desktop or even deep searches. The reader will find the information given above is entirely validated by highly qualified medical researchers at top universities and institutions who are pursuing separate studies of

GSH topics.

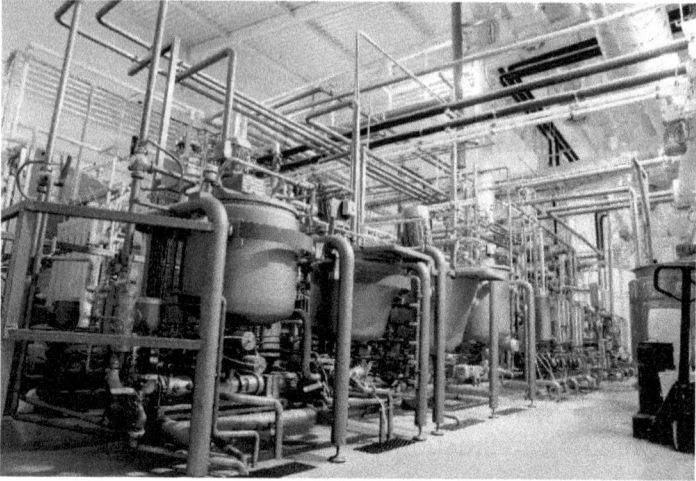

I have simply juxtaposed all these researchers' outcomes, and although GSH, even as the common denominator in Covid-19 research, is not on the low-hanging fruit of vaccines, it would, nonetheless, improve Covid-19 infection and fatality rates considerably while vaccines are still being developed and distributed.

What is also needed is perhaps an independent government lead and a funded national centre for amino, antioxidant and glutathione research, either to continue funding the studies started by academics, or through sponsorship or funding from pharmaceutical companies. Many of the academic clinical researchers cited in this document share this view.

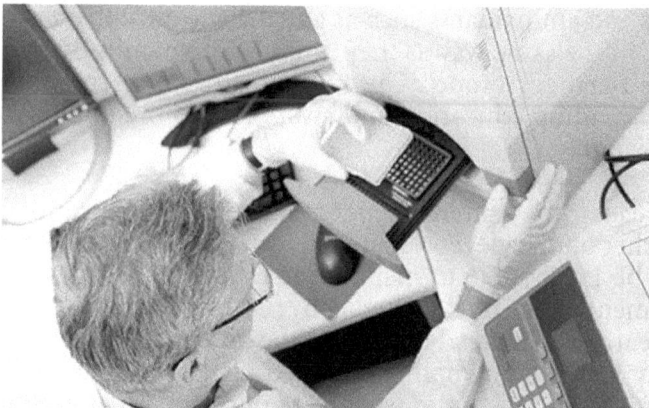

11. A QUICK COVID-19 SUPPLEMENT SOLUTION

The Covid solution is a glutathione (GSH) combination in an oral (or IV) supplement made of free-form amino acids in NAC, GLY and GLU, to assist the synthesis of the greater GSH requirements for a stressed immune system.

It is better to ingest the amino components individually rather than in a manufactured GSH as they will survive the digestive journey better, or the Lipsomal GSH combination should also be considered where available.

The addition of alpha-lipoic acid (ALA) and vitamins E, C, B6, B12, B1 and B2, which are often ineffective unless working in conjunction with amino acids, serve to ensure the efficiency of the synthesised GSH. Vitamins C and E, for instance, aid the immune system by recycling GSH, increasing its availability and resource, a function I expect few readers are aware of.

Patients showing early symptoms should also treat with the above daily supplements containing the full spectrum or at least the essential aminos.

Further treating with mebendazole is advised to remove any helminth parasitic stress on the immune system. All the above are natural products, and Mebendezole in the Ovex version is non-prescription.

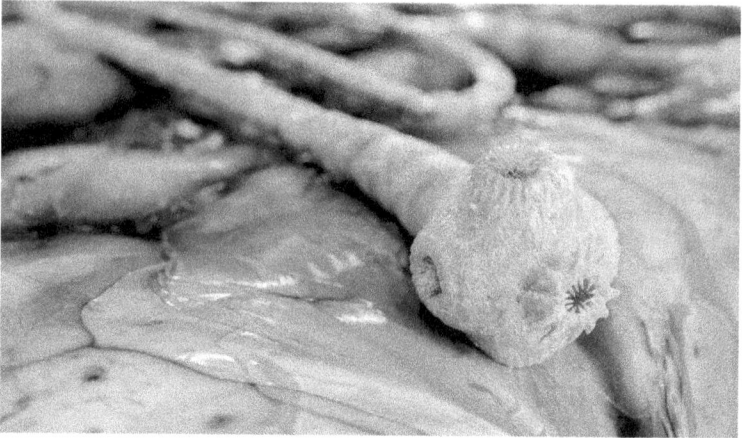

DOSING

Basic Covid-19 amino-based daily supplement

On the basis of the average person's diet containing an average amount of aminos, G & G, a UK manufacturer and distributor of amino acids, suggests that nutritionists prescribe a minimum daily dosage for the free-form aminos, as specified below (free-form in simple terms means 'pre-digested' aminos, formulated to be instantly available for vascular absorption):

- L-cysteine 48mg
- L-glutamine 150mg
- L-glycine 48mg

I would also add a further L-methionine (9mg per day) which, from my observations, is a cysteine-supporting amino.

These dosage suggestions would need to be confirmed by the readers clinician or nutritionist or the supplement vendor, being subject to individual physiology such as prior diet, body weight or allergies.

The above quantities of supplementation are intended for the average healthy body physiology (of a non-vulnerable group) with an average diet that includes a generally balanced amount of aminos present for use. This is a baseline minimum supplementation that should protect the majority of people that are currently healthy, or those with only mild vulnerabilities. It is certainly better than no supplementation for those with identified Covid-19 vulnerabilities.

If Covid-19 symptoms appear, this dosing should be doubled, then trebled on the third day, and maintained until symptoms subside; under a clinician's supervision of course.

This supplementation may prevent a mild Covid-19 illness from developing into a serious or critical illness in the majority of patients. In order to build up the necessary concentration in the body, it should be started, along with any vitamin supplementation necessary, before any symptoms appear.

Calculating the amino acids in your diet

Use this online tool app to calculate the amino acids in different foods:

https://tools.myfooddata.com/nutrient-ranking-tool

Supplementing the GSH amino component through food

Given that this book is about nutrition, we clearly need to look at ways to increase the three aminos of cysteine, glycine and glutamine required through our food. Some people may not wish to use prepared, processed supplements, or may be unable to do so due to future governmental enforcement of prescriptions only for aminos supply

To recap: the body, when under stress from sickness or toxicity, will seek to obtain further stores of the GSH aminos required to synthesise the GSH supplied through our diet. The foods containing the three aminos required are listed below: (RDI =Recommended Daily Intake)

Cysteine (287mg = 100% RDI)

- obtained from chicken and turkey

- for vegetarians: eggs and low-fat yogurt

- for vegans: legumes, peas, couscous and lentils

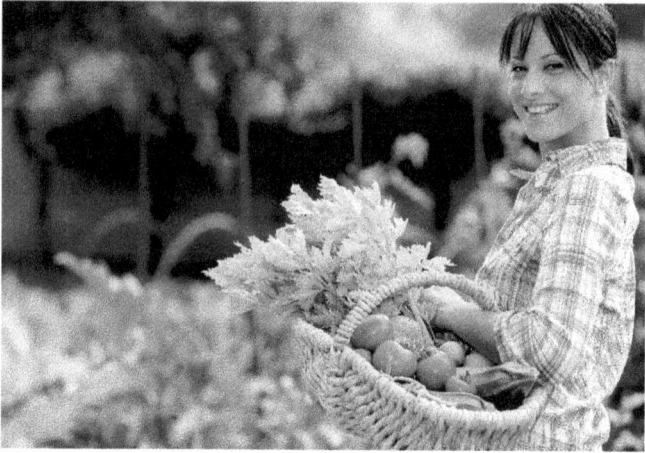

Glycine (no recommended RDI)

- obtained from red meats, turkey, chicken, pork, gelatine salmon

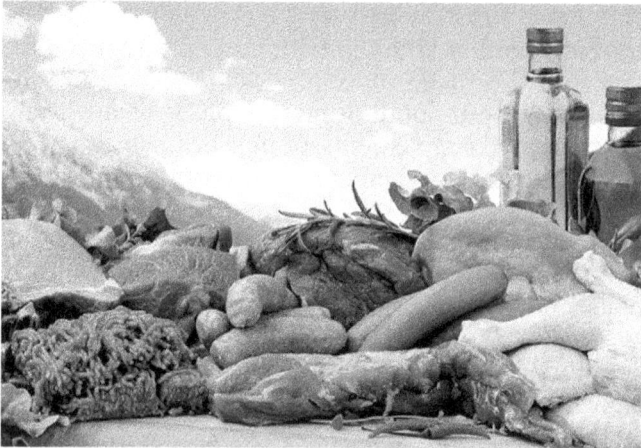

- for vegetarians / vegans: sesame and pumpkin seeds, peanuts and granola

Glutamic acid / glutamine (no recommended RDI)

- obtained from chicken and fish
- for vegetarians: dairy produce
- for vegans: beans, lentils, tofu, spinach and cabbage

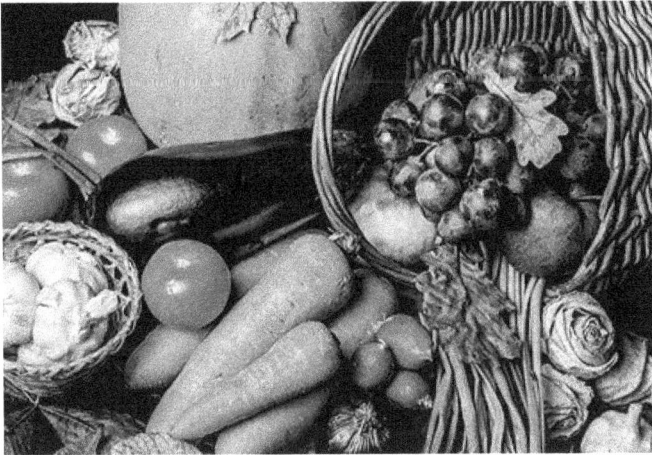

Fast-track or emergency GSH amino components through food

To take the guess work out of such supplementing, or as an alternative to calculating the food amino values on the app mentioned above, for example, or if the relevant fresh foods are not available, the aminos can be obtained in the form of dried foods. Given that non-essential aminos are, in general, simply obtained from proteins, all the amino components above can be obtained from egg white powder or soybean protein powder. The source data for the details below was taken from the US Department of Agriculture website.

Dried egg white powder, glucose reduced 100g (1 cup) provides approximately:

- cysteine, 2.04g
- glutamic acid, 11.5g
- glycine, 3.08g

Soy protein powder 100g (1 cup) provides approximately:

- cysteine, 0.700g
- glutamic acid, 10.8g
- glycine, 2.37g

As you will note, half-a-cup of dried egg white powder or a half cup with equal amounts of soy protein powder and egg-white powder—to bolster the cysteine element—will more than cover the RDI of the amino elements of glutathione synthesis.

Note: The amounts you need should also be discussed with your nutritionist or clinician because the physiology differs between individuals, and he / she would take into account any underlying diseases, medical conditions or allergies. The recommended protein intake is 0.8g per kilogram of body weight per day

Having also examined some pea protein brands, I found them to contain small amounts of cysteine but no glycine or glutamine. If the reader prefers, mixing pea protein with egg-white powder or soy protein powder will provide the complete components.

Research by Engy M. El Morsy et al. reveals that artichoke leaf and artichoke-leaf extract helps—to express it simply to prevent the wastage of GSH. This was proven in rat subjects dosed with paracetamol or analgesic toxicity to stress the GSH supply. I have made artichoke hearts, as a superfood, part of my diet for many years.

I am recommending organic versions of any soya products, as non-organic varieties may have been processed with hexane, which is a hydrocarbon similar to petroleum. Hexane even smells like petrol! I have never been certain why the US FDA approved such a toxic substance used for production of human or animal consumption food, doubtless it was based on proven safe testing.

Plants noted as being complete (essential) aminos (not non-essential or conditional aminos) include quinoa, amaranth grains, spirulina buckwheat and chia seeds. Soya, however, covers the essential, non-essential and conditional amino range required for glutathione supplementing.

Nutrient supplements and plant or egg protein powders generally rely on processed food production processes and should be used as emergency or convenience when traveling or during sickness, for example, or as a means of maintaining nutrient levels when the necessary fresh foods are not available. There is, however, no long-term substitute for obtaining these nutrients from fresh, organic, non-processed food sources.

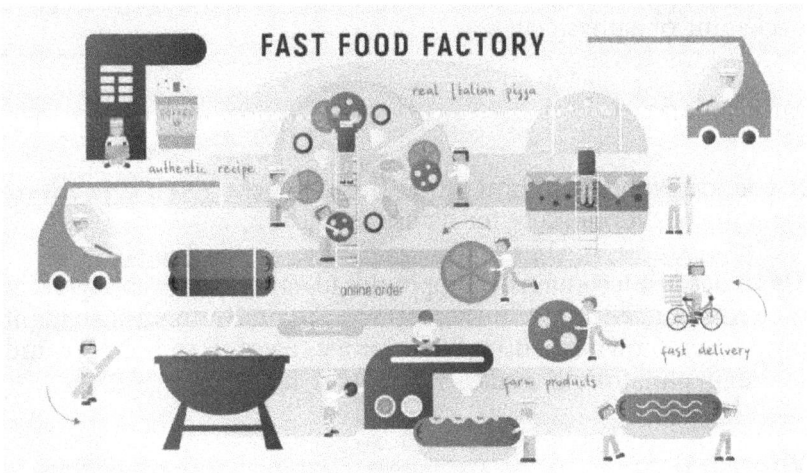

GLUTATHIONE BOOSTERS

Sulphur Rich Foods

Sulphur is at the heart of Glutathione and its synthesis. Sulphur is concentrated in two aminos Cysteine & Methionine so eating Amino protein such as quality Chicken, Beef, Fish or Sulphur containing vegetables such kale, Broccoli, Mustard greens, cauliflower, onions garlic or shallots as or as also mentioned above Pea, Soy & Whey protein providing full amino supplementation covering Cysteine and Methionine

Artichokes and Artichoke Extract

Has recently been found to have positive effect on reducing the loss of Glutathione due to cellular leakage, while this needs more research however current results indicate that it is a viable antioxidant protection for glutathione

Selenium

Selenium is required for the synthesis of Glutathione, and works in conjunction with GSH Avocados Asparagus and Brazil nuts are extremely rich in selenium Note there are upper limits for Selenium Supplementation daily so advice should be sort from the vendors packaging or a physician

Milk Thistle

If you are wondering how Milk Thistle works given it is a long standing traditional cure for illness and health,

This is because it contains 3 compounds together known as Silymarin which is concentrated in the extract. Silymarin has antioxidant properties shown in animal laboratory research to increase and maintain glutathione levels

Vitamin C

This has been covered in other areas if this book given it has the ability not only as a alone anti-oxidant can recycle or "clean" Glutathione

A recap of other Vitamins helpful to Glutathione

The addition of alpha-lipoic acid (ALA) and vitamins E, C, B6, B12, B1 and B2, which are often ineffective unless working in conjunction with amino acids, serve to ensure the efficiency of the synthesised GSH. Vitamins C and E, for instance, aid the immune system by recycling GSH, increasing its availability and resource, a function I expect few readers are aware of.

Artichokes Asparagus and Avocados have been long standing part of my diet which I view as superfoods. As mentioned in this book, excessive Alcohol consumption has a serious derogatory effect on Glutathione levels and good Sleep and moderate exercise has a positive effect.

In my view poor education, limited research, dysfunctional diet, defective nutrition through factory farming and food processing with non-organic ingredients not containing the necessary dietary support for Glutathione and antioxidants, is at the heart of poor Antioxidant levels and immune system capability and capacity to resist Covid 19 and other virus and bacterial infections.

These issues deny our bodies ability to have a normalised immune system especially with age. On the basis that vaccines require a normalised immune system It may take a conscious decision by the individual too pursue a diet along with nutritional supplementation to boost our bodies natural immune defences and reduce the reliance on prescription pharmaceutical remedies

12. GLUTATHIONE DOSING IN CRITICAL CARE.
(Section Relevant to Clinicians)

Research has shown that with 1000mg per day orally ingested, prepared GSH can take up to six months to establish regular levels in patients with depleted levels. At least 3000mg per day should be considered for a depleted subject to reduce the saturation time to under a month. Additionally, a chelation doctor should be consulted. See page 61 for the description of a doctor's successful prescription on a critical care Covid-19 patient.

Liposomal GSH or S-acetyl glutathione (for oral administration) should be administered either in line with the manufacturer's dosing recommendation or with the 3 individual GSH amino components taken separately.

Homeostasis

Also important is keeping the patient in a state of fluids Homeostasis by use of blood PH monitoring and supplements containing necessary mineral ions support such as Potassium, Sodium, calcium, which may be found in part in digestive antacids such as Alka Seltzer Gold

L- or N-acetyl amino acids

There has been much debate on the ability of N-acetyl to be absorbed in water and to pass through the digestive system easily, compared to the L version, which is more bioavailable at the cellular level after passing through the digestive system, given that the N acetyl version has to be 'unpacked' and converted and is essentially a precursor of cysteine.

According to a detailed study from the Mustafa Kemal University Turkey:

"One of the main reasons why NAC is preferred over cysteine in vivo experimental systems is that NAC does not become oxidized easily in the intestinal fluid, whereas cysteine is rapidly oxidized and converted to cysteine, whose absorption requires exchange with Glutamate. [19] This result further indicates that cysteine is more resistant to oxidation in a physiological buffer than in intestinal fluid. Our results suggest that cysteine, which is less frequently used in experimental systems, may provide faster and better results than expected from the well-recognised NAC that is more widely used, especially in the in-vitro experimental systems. Cysteine is more readily available for the cells when compared with NAC."

Further comment is beyond the scope of this document, and the full study needs to be read in the context of the amino usage. Clearly, both acetyl types will play their part in the GSH synthesis. I note that NAC it is also used for COPD patient treatment by Dr Pangrazzi at the University of Innsbruck, [7] and it appears to be a favorite for respiratory care. As I am not a clinician, however, this choice is clearly one to be made at that level and with the appropriate medical resources

Initial laboratory studies on S-acetyl glutathione (S GSH) suggest it is more robust in oral administration and vascular transport, and will raise the glutathione levels in cells in greater volume than non-acetylated glutathione. S GSH is a version of the readily available reduced, or L-glutathione. Further clinical study is needed for additional proof, however.

Injectable GSH is manufactured and available for seriously ill patients, although research has indicated that it lasts at full-strength for only 4 hours or so. It would therefore need to be administered to these subjects through an IV drip or by dosing 6 times per day, with regular blood tests to measure the concentrations.

Helminth parasite condition

Should the clinician wish to apply my recommendation of relieving further immune system strain resulting from any worm infestations causing immune system actions to rid them, by the parasites own reported GSH usage and the toxicity and asymptomatic infections by using Vermox or similar prescriptions, care should be taken with seriously ill patients. The effect of Herxhiemer or 'parasite die-off' may temporarily add toxicity to the body in larger infestations. (I think many Clinicians are perplexed by the antivaxxers use of anti parasite medication, it is valid to a degree but on its own is unlikely to totally ensure immunity, in any circumstances Helminth Parasites should not be tolerated in any healthy body and I wonder how many times Clinicians do routinely prescribe given the extremely high average numbers of those infected without symptoms)

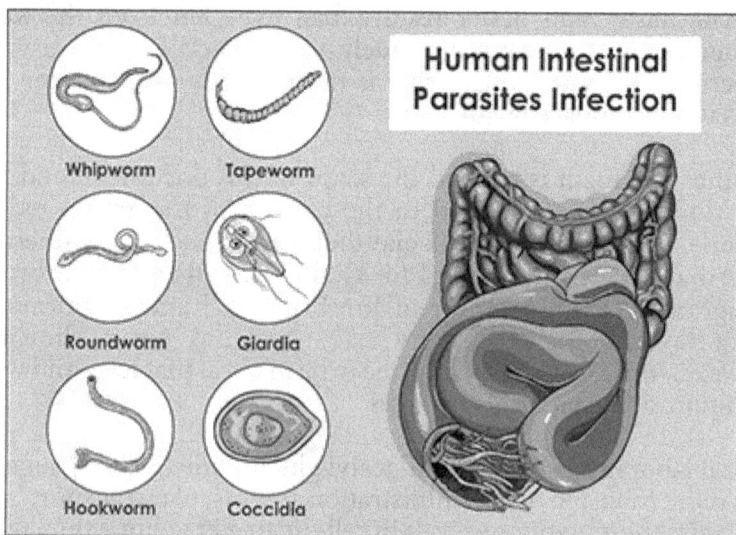

Human Intestinal Parasites Infection

Whipworm   Tapeworm

Roundworm   Giardia

Hookworm   Coccidia

L-cysteine and L-acetyl cysteine dosing in critical care

With L-cysteine (CYS) (or NAC acetylcysteine), the daily amounts required are quite small with a minimum of 50mg for daily supplementing in healthy patients, as the patient will still be obtaining aminos from food if they are still eating normally (see page 24 for food amino calculator).

The body's normal usage of cysteine under normal circumstances from a well and functioning body is, according to WHO, around 1g per day, so supplementation will be necessary if nutrition is absent or reduced, and with an additional dosage to provide the additional requirement of GSH in sickness, as mentioned above.

Cysteine is not as abundant in the body as glycine and glutamine, and is effective in respiratory support on its own. Cysteine could, therefore, be the primary weak link and should be first port of call in any treatment.

The University of Michigan Health System states: "the following daily doses were used in clinical trials evaluating NAC for various conditions: Bronchitis, 400 mg to 600 mg; chronic obstructive pulmonary disease, 200 mg three times a day; angina, 600 mg three times a day; gastritis, 1,000 mg; HIV/AIDS, 800 mg". [20]

Possibly as a life-threatening immune system failure, Covid-19 dosing should be similar to that for HIV initially.

Lai et al. reported that higher levels of NAC at 1200mg twice daily quickly increased glutathione levels during chronic inflammatory disease. Dr Horowitz's prescription on states NAC 1200mg TLD.

L-glycine dosing in critical care

The amounts of glycine supplementation required are quite small: less than 50mg daily if the nutrition is already balanced. Similar to glutamine below, it is more abundant in the body than NAC.

Dosages of oral glycine used in clinical studies for therapeutic purposes range from 2 to 6g daily. Note that taking glycine along with clozapine might reduce the effectiveness of clozapine. Dosages for this condition are very large, at 3 to 9g daily. (superfoodssceintificresearch.com) care should be taken in respect of patients with liver damage with high dosing and further advice should be sought.

L-glutamine dosing in critical care

Glutamine supplements vary in dosages from 500 to 5000mg. Available in pill or powder form, this 'dispensable' amino (one synthesised by the body) can become a 'conditional' one provided from food or supplementation. Athletes routinely use large quantities of glutamine for muscle repair, and given that the lungs are muscles, it can be helpful in treating respiratory disease. The dosage can be increased depending on the level of damage.

Dr Michael Janson suggests 1000–2000mg twice daily, although he notes that higher doses may benefit some people. [21] Jesse L. Hanley and Nancy Deville recommend a 3500mg dose of L-glutamine from one to three times a day. Doses of 500mg daily are generally considered safe, according to University of Maryland Medical Center (Livestrong.com). [22]

L-methionine dosing in critical care

Although not part of our GSH tri-peptide amino package, methionine, as a supporting amino for cysteine, can be considered for inclusion. The recommended daily intake of L-methionine, according to WHO, is 13mg per kilogram of body weight; that is, 988mg for someone weighing 12 stones. Guidance should be sought from a qualified clinical nutritionist for greater volumes.

Continuing care

I repeat that all the above aminos (CYS, GLU, GLY) are 'conditional' amino acids, so the body will scavenge for them from food ingestion once internal synthesis is insufficient for the immune system to function properly, not only during illness but also throughout the recuperation period when the immune system is still under stress. A good diet and dietary supplement program should be established in consultation with a qualified medical nutritionist. L-glutamine should be continued in large quantities.

To assist with lung repair, L-glutamine GLU and GSH also continue to assist with any re-infections and inflammation in the brain caused by Covid-19, which may continue to give 'brain fog' issues in recuperating patients.

Alpha-lipoic acid

The ability of alpha-lipoic acid (ALA) to enhance the glutathione function—and assist in recycling GSH—leads to improved levels of GSH in cases of deficiency. Most known diseases show glutathione deficiencies, especially in their chronic state. Recommended dosages of supplemental lipoic acid are 100 to 200mg per day.

Linoleic acid and conjugated linoleic acid

Linoleic acid (LA) is not to be confused with lipoic acid; they simply share a similar name and abbreviation. As mentioned earlier, narrative studies confirm that conjugated linoleic acid (CLA) up-regulates GSH synthesis, so supplementation should be considered. As CLA is a well-known and commonly used supplement, Covid-19 patients should be given CLA while further research is ongoing.

13. TESTING - A SIMPLE METHOD TO IDENTIFY THOSE INFECTED OR AT RISK OF INFECTION

It appears that addressing GSH and CYS deficiencies is critical to managing immune system strain. Daily blood or saliva testing may therefore identify GSH depletion from illness or diet deficiencies in those who may be infected or are at risk of infection through poor diet or supplementation, as detailed on page 34.

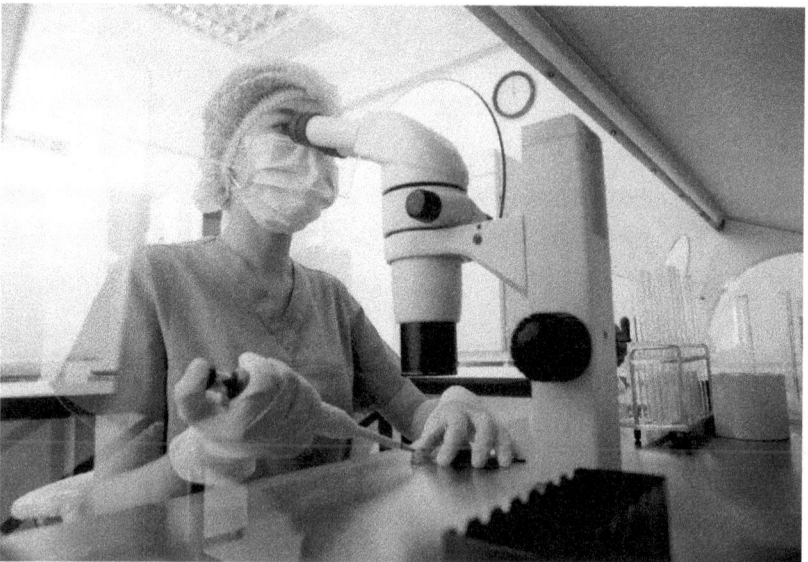

Low-blood levels of GSH can be a sign that the body is under stress, is fighting an infection or is simply at risk, either due to a poor diet or an underlying illness. Glutathione levels can be checked through tests such as 'RBC glutathione', which shows the level of glutathione in red blood cells (RBCs). Although continued low GSH indicates a critical vulnerability to Covid-19, this is rarely measured in routine patient blood tests.

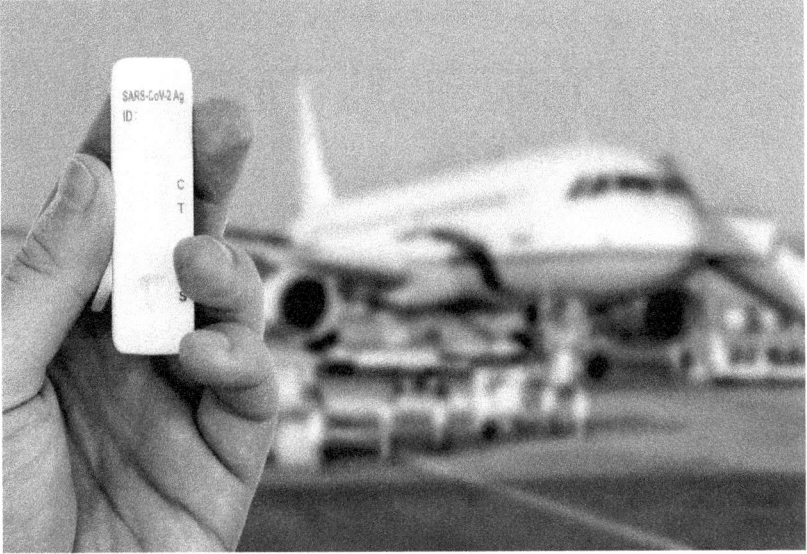

14. THREE DUCKS IN A ROW

From the narrative above, we can see that Covid-19 needs:

- a vulnerability that reduces GSH or cysteine synthesis
- a poor diet that does not sustain cysteine and GSH synthesis when required 'conditionally', and is not supplemented to compensate
- a lifestyle that hampers GSH synthesis and promotes exposure to infection

It has frequently been asked: "How did this fit, young, super-healthy and athletic individual succumb to Covid-19?" It is no surprise to me that the rigorous excessive exercise associated with vanity body-beautiful pursuits such as weightlifting or marathon running—especially without professional dietary supervision—can deplete the amino levels, especially glutamine, and can cause muscle damage, oxidative stress and further depletion of GSH.

Added to this, the Gym and exercise based protein-rich power diets and supplements normally focussed on BCA (Branch Chain Amino acids) can fail to provide balanced amino nutrition, as well as the low-calorie vanity dieting followed by slimmer's, also exacerbate depletion, both in substance and in volume.

Another factor, furthermore, is the mistaken belief that good health is based totally on potentially compromised synthesised anhydrous vitamins. Also, in an internal gym environment, contact with other, seemingly fit yet vulnerable, individuals can heighten the chances of infection. Granted, the fit, young body may recover more quickly as, without other physical immunity-mechanism encumbrances, it will bounce back more easily.

Exercise should be performed in moderation and remembering that a doctor would advise against exercising during illness. Indeed, others exercising in the gym may be infected, sick or vulnerable, perhaps falsely assuming that the more they exercise, the healthier they will be, while they are actually creating an infectious situation potentially compromising the immune by over or extremely excessive vanity exercising increasing Oxidative stress and reducing GSH levels

15. THE UK – ONE OF THE MOST VULNERABLE POPULATION IN 2020

Population 60 million: 90,000 Covid-19 deaths as at Jan 2021

Putting all this narrative together, alongside the relevant health statistics, one of the most vulnerable Covid-19 models might be a male British citizen, aged 55+, who is severely obese (BMI 35 +) African American, an alcoholic, possibly a diabetic or borderline diabetic and may also have an invisible gluten intolerance, as well as helminth parasitic worms and mercury amalgam dental fillings. Further characteristics of vulnerability are, a low income and low-food budget, a poorly balanced diet without adequate supplementation with vitamins and amino acids and an underlying respiratory disease. The model would possibly also be a smoker of tobacco or narcotics and would live in a densely populated inner city or industrial area with poor air quality.

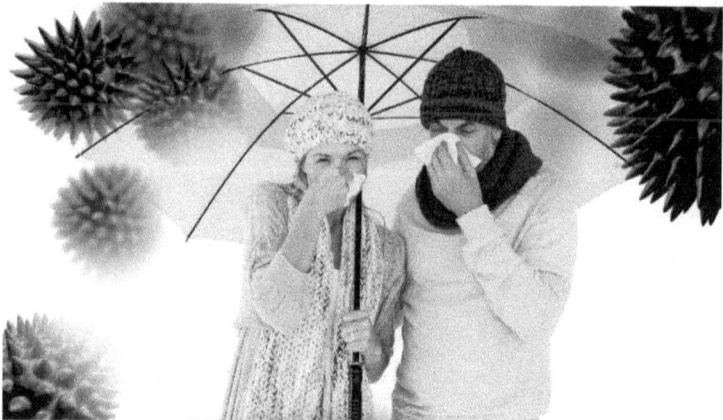

Possibly why the mortuaries may have been full of this model type especially in the UK (and US).

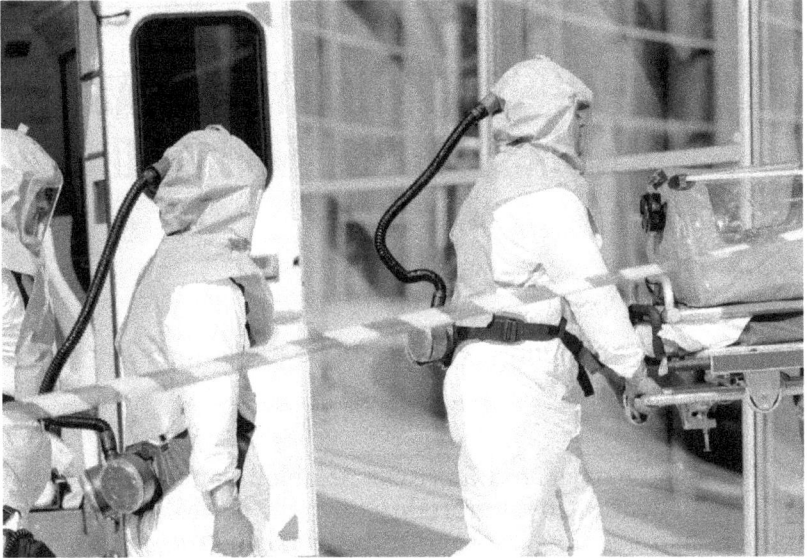

16. JAPAN – POTENTIALLY THE LEAST VULNERABLE POPULATION 2020

Population 120 million: 4000 Covid-19 deaths as at Jan 2021

The population of Japan comprises a notable anomaly in having an exceptionally low Covid mortality rate. The Covid record shows higher than average recovery and mortality rates for its huge population size, even with large numbers concentrated in dense city environments. With twice the population of the UK, Japan shows only a fraction of the UK's mortality rate.

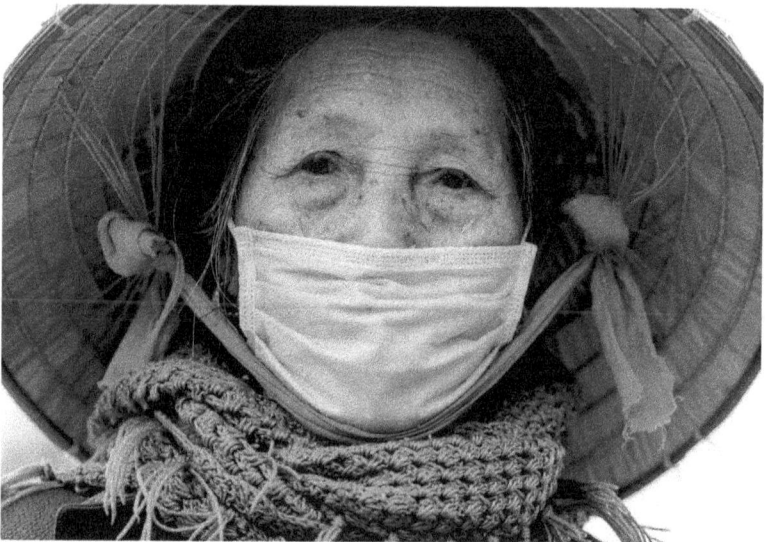

So why is Japan's resilience disproportionate? It simply has an exceptionally healthy amino-inclusive diet that gives the population reduced mortalities—not only for Covid—but also in other areas such as heart disease and cancer.

Could the reason also be because Mitsubishi is the only global enterprise, I could find that, through its subsidiaries, funds research into glutathione, and that the population in Japan supplements with glutathione more commonly than elsewhere? Further research is clearly required here and is possibly being conducted already.

Covid-19 protection in Japan will be due, at least in part, to the diet. Avoiding any fanciful popular speculation without evidence, let us take a scientific perspective. The Japanese consume 2 items in far greater abundance than populations in the west: soya beans and soy sauce. Soy sauce is basically an 'amino soup', especially as it is extremely rich in one of our 3 GSH amino components, cysteine, in addition to methionine, another supportive amino of cysteine in GSH synthesis.

As cysteine is the most important amino, particularly as it is effective alone in respect of respiratory illness, and also, importantly, it does not occur in food as abundantly as its two GSH amino counterparts. Just a cup of many soya-based products contains around 287mg of cysteine and provides the RDI, which perhaps explains the reason the Japanese diet promotes immunity against much critical illness.

As a conditional amino, cysteine will be required from food when synthesis is under strain from serious illness. Can soy sauce help prevent the escalation of Covid-19 infection? Yes it can, far-fetched as this may sound. The evidence suggests so and gives further proof for the amino-acid deficient diet argument.

17. RELATIONSHIP BETWEEN VITAMIN D AND GSH - & WHY VIT D ?

If we need further proof, we need look no further than the clinical research published in 2020 in the Journal of Steroid Biochemistry confirming that vitamin D administered in high doses can reduce ICU admission by a staggering 97 percent. [23]

I *do not believe* this startling claim for the reasons stated as follows. If we look at the researchers' recommended dosing of 104,400 k IUs on day 1, and 53,200 IUs on days 3 and 7, and then 53,200 IUs once a week thereafter, we can see that a simple vitamin D deficiency at these levels can hardly be the only root cause of the progression to critical Covid-19 infections. Such levels are hardly likely to ever be found in any normal diet in the majority of the world's population that do not develop critical Covid-19 infection or in those developing only mild symptoms. Here one assumes that such high doses are being used therapeutically for vitamin D's steroid capability.

After all there may be no actual vitamin D deficiency in sunny countries yet we still see high infection rates and critical care admissions in such countries.

So why is this high supplementation so necessary with patients on the brink of critical care who are clearly then seriously deficient in vitamin D after Covid-19 infection?

Well, we are back to glutathione and a study entitled 'GSH and Vitamin D Interaction', which states that "GSH stimulates vitamin D regulatory and glucose metabolism and supplementation of GSH" in a novel approach to treating 25-Hydroxy vitamin D deficiency. [24]

The study goes on to suggest that it is indeed a GSH deficiency itself that causes or contributes to the vitamin D deficiency. The lack of

GSH to stimulate and regulate vitamin D actually prevents the body from utilising the steroidal effect of vitamin D in its immune system arsenal, and so extreme emergency supplementation of the depleted vitamin D is required at the critical illness stage.

Once again, the common denominator deficient in Covid-19 critical infection outcomes is glutathione and, of course, its three precursor amino acids as a tri-peptide.

18. LONG COVID

I will not go into too much detail as this section is worthy of a separate white paper, but I will simply record my own experiences in treating the post-Covid-19 residual effects in my own illness.

Brain fog

The large quantities of GSH normally present in the brain serve as an anti-inflammatory, and it is my belief that post-Covid brain fog is caused by residual inflammation and depleted GSH. As the virus enters mainly from ACE 2 receptors in the sinuses, adjacent to the brain, the infection and subsequent inflammation of this organ is not an unreasonable assumption. This would explain the signature painful migraine-like headaches as symptoms of the Covid-19 infection that are caused by brain inflammation.

When fighting the infection, a body perhaps already deficient in GSH could be more seriously depleted in post-infection or even simply to reduce the cranial brain inflammation. In this case, continued supplementation of GSH should be considered. I found that liposomal GSH taken twice daily cured this condition for me within weeks.

Breathlessness

I continued amino full spectrum and GSH oral ingestion with additional L-glutamine, on the basis that glutamine is used by athletes for muscle and tissue repair after exercise. The work of the lungs is performed by the intercostal, neck and abdominal muscles that may also have suffered during Covid, which may explain any chest pains in post-Covid patients. I continued oxygen therapy using an oxygen concentrator machine at Fi02 95% 3 litres minimum

(FiO2 is the fraction of O2 percentage in an air mix) for 3 hours daily overnight and found a return to normal breathing fitness within two weeks. Further, dosing of asthmatic preventer inhaler steroid therapeutics such as Clenil Modulite is also recommended, and this yielded rapid results in my case.

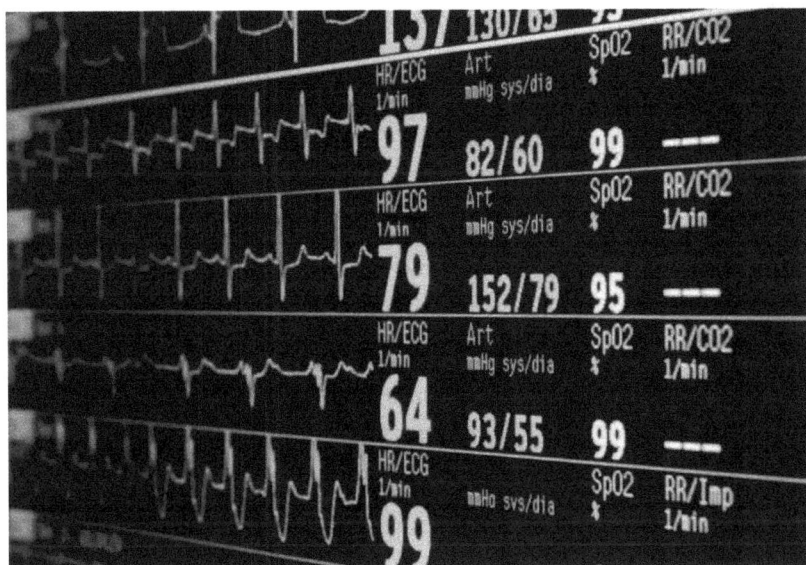

Rhinosinusitis and lost sense of smell due to olfactory nerve damage

This was the dual result I had from many years of suffering from rhinosinusitis, which gave rise to the sleep Apnea condition. It became much worse after my Covid-19 infection and overnight monitoring showed a lower SP02 as well as the more serious sleep apnea episodes with O2 below 90 percent.

In treating the loss of smell, I sprayed liquid GSH (Brand: Results RNA ACG Glutathione) into my nostrils in the evening once my nose was dry from the oxygen concentrator and nasal Canalula; applying FI 02 of 95 percent at 3 litres minimum for 3 hours per night, for 3 days. I also applied liquid GSH to the nasal cavities each session.

Within 3 days, my long-term rhinosinusitis had disappeared, and I regained my sense of smell. My SpO2 levels increased, the sleep apnea episodes decreased, and my nasal passages were free and clear.

It is to be noted that pure high concentrations of O2, 100% ideally, applied locally can, in many instances, directly kill a virus or bacteria on contact with the gas, or it can oxygenate the cells to repair. The combination of liquid GSH and 95% FIO2 proved to be a cure for both afflictions.

During this period, I continued oral ingestion of full-spectrum aminos plus liposomal and L-glutathione in its combined precursor component forms.

It is important to note that orally ingested L-glutamine, as mentioned above, is useful for muscle and tissue repair. This may have been a component in the nerve repair but cannot be confirmed.

Hypertension (High Blood Pressure)

Alarming rates of Hypertension (high blood pressure) have and are now being observed, during and after the COVID pandemics, and during 2022 especially in the US the US CDC (Centre for Disease control) reported a staggering unsurpassed increase in hypertension in the population.

Given the Covid infection enters the body through the ACE 2 receptors which are bio sensors that measure for instance body temperature, Blood PH and indeed Blood pressure to keep the body in Homeostasis, a self-regulated monitored state, perhaps COVID has damaged these sensors, the exact reason is unknown and needs further research.

What is known is that most of the world populations consume an alarming amount of Salt in food especially in processed food often more than 10 times the RDA (Cheese being a particular culprit) and very little Potassium. Too much salt and too little Potassium is a deadly embrace for hypertension. Perhaps COVID damage will no longer allow the body to tolerate or regulate such in the diet so remove excess Salt from diet by reading food packaging and eat a banana a day (subject to allergies) each banana around 400mgs of potassium or use Potassium supplements - the RDA of Potassium being 3,600mgs, buy yourself a blood pressure monitor or see a physician and report high or elevated findings especially over 140 SYS (Systolic) or any hypertension symptoms urgently to your clinician as you may require specific medication as well as diet change to control this potentially deadly condition.

Studies have linked Glutathione use to help reduce Blood pressure in people with say Coronary artery diseases, patients receiving Glutathione saw an increase in blood vessel diameter, and studies from Thibaud Damy et al [29] in their studies are quoted as saying that "Blood Glutathione tests may be an interesting bio marker to detect asymptomatic patients with structural arterial problems". However, in this instance I would refer anyone to consult with their clinician in the first instance before supplementing with Glutathione given the cause of hypertension may be unknown.

19. THE UNIVERSITY OF KURSK STUDY: PROOF OF CONCEPT

In his report on the endogenous deficiency o f g lutathione, D r Polonikov notes that "Since the antiviral effect o f G lutathione is nonspecific, there is reason to believe that glutathione is also active against SARS-CoV-2. Therefore, restoration of glutathione levels in Covid-19 patients would be a promising approach for the management of the novel coronavirus SARS-CoV-2. Notably, long-term oral administration of N-acetyl cysteine has already been tested as an effective preventive measure against respiratory viral infections. N-acetyl cysteine is widely available, safe, and cheap and could be used in an 'off-label' manner. Moreover, parenteral injection of NAC or reduced glutathione (GSH is more bioavailable than NAC) could be an efficient therapy for Covid-19 patients with serious illness." [25]

The days described for the recovery or disappearance of COVID 19 symptoms are in direct relationship to the vascular GSH levels in respective patients, reduced by their pre existing conditions. This is positive proof of the direct relationship of GSH levels to the severity of illness experienced by COVID 19 patients. The link to the clinical evidence from Dr Polonikov's study given in his work is at [25] in the references section of this book.

Relationship between GSH and Covid-19 severity and recovery

"Glutathione deficiency in Covid-19 patients with serious illness may also be a result of decreased consumption of fresh vegetables and fruits (especially during winter and spring seasons), which contributes to over 50 percent of dietary glutathione intake", reports Dr Polonikov. "The hypothesis suggests that SARS-CoV-2 virus poses a danger only for people with endogenous glutathione deficiency, regardless [of] which … the factors [of] aging, chronic disease comorbidity, smoking or some others were responsible for this deficit", he adds. [25]

Polinikov also promotes the study by Dr R. I. Horowitz, as I do, which further confirms Polinikov's findings. As respected, qualified clinicians, in their common qualified findings from separate interventional trials, they both corroborate on the efficacy of GSH detailed in this book and its precursors in treating Covid-19.[26]

Further, Dr Horowitz states that glutathione precursors NAC and alpha-lipoic acid, together with oral and IV GSH may, therefore, represent a novel treatment approach for addressing *cytokine storm syndrome* and respiratory distress in patients with Covid-19 pneumonia. [26] His successful alternative prescription for a critical care patient not responding to antibiotics (Amoxi Clav) follows:

"Reduced, liposomal glutathione was added to her antibiotic regimen (Amoxi Clav) along with 50 mg of zinc and 1-g TID (*3 Times Day*) of Vitamin C. The patient was given 2000 mg of l-Glutathione PO *(Orally)* all at once with 2 Alka seltzer gold, (for acid indigestion) along with alpha-lipoic acid 600 mg, and N-acetylcysteine 1200 mg." [27]

The patient seaw an immediate improvement described as "being able to breathe better and having more energy, within an hour of use. After administration of the Glutathione, the cough resolved and she was able to sleep through the night for the first time since the onset of illness, despite having been on her antibiotic regimen for several days."

Note the use of Alka Selzer Gold. It is important to ensure stomach acidity is not excessive and that blood PH (Acid / Alkaline balance) remains as neutral as possible. When the blood PH becomes too high the body will rob the kidneys of minerals and nutrients to use to correct the PH condition which may deplete some of the prescriptive supplementations. The term Homeostasis is state of steady regularised chemical conditions of say the fluid balances and body temperature including the PH of extracellular fluid and the optimal concentrations of Sodium, Potassium and Calcium ions. Potassium and Sodium Minerals are within Alka Seltzer Gold, this enables the immune system to better perform within state of Homeostasis.

Both Polonikov and Horowitz's sample studies and the component parts of their prescriptions are validated in my own lengthy research and observations.

The prescription components mentioned need further government-backed interventional clinical trials with a view to widespread release. [27] In fact, these trials should be fast-tracked as a precaution against the shortfall in vaccine efficacy for any new variant strains, as the evidence is overwhelming that GSH and it precursor components, especially cysteine, reduce or eliminate the critical effects of Covid-19.

The full studies by Polonikov and Horowitz can be obtained from the web addresses given in the referance section.

20. SUMMARY

What we can do now to reduce Covid-19 infection and mortality rates

In terms of mortality, I am working to assess the percentage of Covid-19 fatalities from, for instance, the terminally ill smokers of approximately 70,000 annually in the UK that would have died of respiratory failure in any case, and this group would, of course, have been highly susceptible. In other words, how far did this group influence the fatality statistics negatively?

For the majority of the population, a supplement containing full-spectrum (all 20) amino acids is already available over the counter at pharmacies (or through Amazon). Taken twice daily, it will provide a more robust first wave immune system defence and reduce the escalation of critical cases by millions.

Supplementing with full-spectrum amino acids is preferable to taking the more popular essential aminos (those obtained from the diet). When the non-essential aminos (those produced by the body) are depleted in Covid-19 critical cases, the supplement provides a further source of GSH tri-peptide when its component non-essential aminos become conditional and are scavenged from food.

Dosing should be in accordance with the manufacturer's or distributor's recommendation, or as specified in the section for clinicians above.

All serious or critical care Covid-19 patients should have a glutathione red blood cell test to ensure at least the minimum recommended RBC 1.6 mmol/l is supplemented immediately if needed.

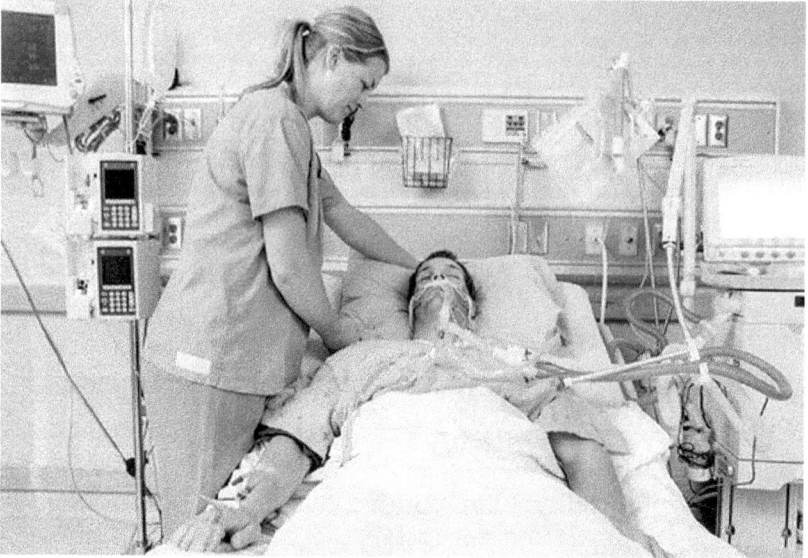

Covid-19 critical care patients should be placed on OP or IV GSH of at least three doses per day, and seriously ill patients on oral liposomal or S-acetyl glutathione, CYS (or NAC), Glutamine (GLU), and GLY supplement (or as recommended in Dr Horowitz's prescription above (see page 61).

Among vulnerable groups, even currently healthy individuals should take full-spectrum amino acids as nutritional supplements 2–4 times per day.

All groups should refrain from excessive alcohol intake and not exceed the government's recommended 3 units per day; supplementing with full-spectrum or essential amino acids after each drinking session and reducing to less than 9 units per week.

Importantly, amino supplements cost very little and are more effective than just vitamin supplementation alone (vitamins may often be ineffective unless complemented by amino supplementation), as already followed in the daily regime of vast majorities of the world population.

Future immunity from Covid-19 by virtue of having had the virus in mild form, may not, therefore, be guaranteed if the patient changes their dietary habits and reduces their amino or GSH capacity. This may result in only a mild IgM immune response in a subsequent infection or even an IgG in the first instance, due the immune system's lower ability to respond effectively.

Can it be that Covid-19 has gone from being a relatively harmless flu to a critical illness threatening the majority of the world's population—particularly the vulnerable groups—simply because of a dietary deficiency? Can diet alone render those that are vulnerable to critical Covid-19 illness, especially in terms of poor amino nutrition when the body requires more glutathione or L-cysteine, glycine and glutamine, than synthesis or diet provide? The answer is yes. The evidence from scientific research and the human test trials detailed above confirm this is the case.

A perfect storm can therefore brew from a few small and seemingly unimportant factors, and conversely, taking a few natural substances and carefully juxtaposing them can quell the storm and create the perfect cure.

Importantly, if the vaccines fail, either in the short- or long-term due to new variant mutations of the virus, or if some patients usually have adverse effects from vaccines, the immune system is likely to adapt much more quickly to new mutations than the labs can create new vaccines. This will only be the case, however, if the immune system and its principle defence mechanisms of GSH and NAC are supported through supplementation and diet.

Governments need to fast-track deeper clinical studies into the supplementation of amino acids, glutathione and cysteine without delay, as experts are saying that further pandemic viruses may be on the way. A fully functioning immune system may therefore serve as a vital fire break until vaccines are developed.

At the same time, governments should also fund and back a PR awareness campaign to inform the public of the amino acids, glutathione and antioxidant supplementation that could be essential for their health. This can be done in the same way that vitamin usage is promoted. The large demand that would follow would give commercial viability and encourage the pharmaceutical industry to pursue production and research; thereby supporting doctors in the field both with prescriptive education and with approved amino- and antioxidant-based products.

Clear research links excessive alcohol consumption with impaired immune system performance in Covid-19 patients, due to the effect of alcohol in suppressing the vital antioxidant GSH. Perhaps the world is not economically or politically ready to impose another prohibition on alcohol as did the US for 13 long years, immediately after the Spanish flu of 1918–1919 – a coincidence? Nutritionists were already warning of a breakdown in nutrition during and after the First World War, as the Spanish flu was coming to an end. Was the Prohibition an attempt to prevent another pandemic? If this was so, the US never stated it and no other nation followed its example by introducing a prohibition on alcohol—ostensibly for reasons of social morality—but regardless, the alcohol available on the black market made the Prohibition an utter farce.

Quite possibly, we have reached a point where the hubris of human technology—ignored at our peril—is finally tumbling world economies and causing havoc to world health. The rarity of a balanced and organic diet that provides the humble natural amino and its antioxidants, synthesized normally, is among the effects.

Perhaps we can all pray that if any good can come from this crisis, it is the wake-up call we need, to protect not only the global environment, but also the environment of the human body. Perhaps nature is teaching us a lesson we will not forget.

It should be noted at time of writing that, curiously, the US FDA appears to be banning or restricted non-prescription sales of NAC in October 2021. This common amino acid, which makes up part of all protein in the human body, is essential to the synthesis of glutathione in our first-line immune defence. Is this a precursor to allowing pharmaceutical companies a commercial monopoly on a natural amino acid that is an effective prevention—and cure—for Covid-19, after all this time has passed and billions have been spent on vaccines, not to mention the millions that have died.

In 2020, I was invited to submit my findings on the subject of glutathione to the UK Government Covid Therapeutics Advisory Panel (UK CTAP group). I did not submit it then, however, because I felt this research would not be taken seriously until the efficacy of vaccinations was known, UK CTAP was subsequently dissolved with little advance notice in September 2021. Given this I was unable to submit after waiting for the first-year outcomes of vaccines to be known and this was badly timed just before the Omicron variant swept into town and infections surged. However it does look like vaccines did their job at least in part. However many vaccinated patients did suffer hospitalisation or death and perhaps we can now consider that diet and nutrition and reduction of alcohol consumption along with routine clinical monitoring of patients

Glutathione levels may further reduce hospitalisation, death and increase the future effectiveness of vaccines.

I do not wish to criticise in any way the use of vaccines along with any recommended boosters, but wish to show that it is vital to the ensure the immune system is—at the same time—functioning efficiently and is properly nourished in order to face and fully respond to a viral attack, which may in turn reduce the long term need for vaccines and boosters as new variants emerge. We can assume perhaps that the vaccines are designed to work most effectively with a normalised well-nourished immune system

It has, however, always been my assertion that giving a human with a poorly nourished immune system a vaccine, which simply put, guides the immune system in terms of the nature of the virus is and how to attack it, is like giving a group of soldiers a map showing the position of the enemy and detailing their strengths and vulnerabilities, but without providing any food or water or any bullets for their guns, then expecting them to enter a series of battles and defeat the enemy.

Amino Acids, Glutathione, Antioxidants and indeed nutrition's importance to human health and longevity is a matter of education, and I hope in some way that this book triggers action or thought leadership towards Education of same - at all levels whether at an individual level or a Governmental, Institutional or Corporate level

On the basis of solid peer reviewed clinical evidence that the Human master antioxidant Glutathione reduces per year on a linear scale, from age 20, largely regardless of individual physiology, so that by the age 60 It is at the WHO defined safe minimum level unless supplemented or reinforced by an appropriate diet. Should Clinicians be considering routine supplementation once confirmed by blood tests?

Finally as I said in the beginning this book was written in as simple language as possible to be generally understood by all, both the layperson, the clinician, general practice Doctor or a medical researcher. My final word for you if you are a non-clinician reading this book is to take clinician's or nutritionist advice and then go ahead and assist your immune system with the right nutrients, nutrition diet and supplements, given a basic understanding of Amino bioscience and its effect on your body immune system you may have gained from this book, it's your way to positively, healthily and sensibly effect the health performance of your body for the better, to feel better and be ill less often and perhaps live longer.

If you are young and if it sounds more fun it may be easier, to think of it as "Bio Hacking" and may help promote you to more interest and study. If you are a Clinician or Health professional, I hope this book points you in the right direction and promotes further study or consultation on the subject particularly of Glutathione and the importance of Amino acids in even general health.

For the layperson non-professional clinician I repeat again, take what you have read in this book to a consultation with your doctor, clinical advisor or nutritionist. After all, I do not know the reader's personal physiology, their medical history, weight or any underlying conditions, allergies or existing dietary or nutritional preferences. Good luck and best wishes with supporting your immune system.

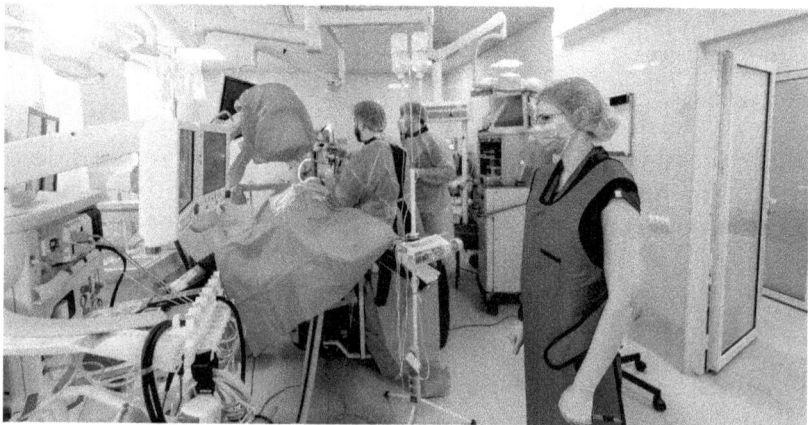

www.friendbiotech.com

21. References & credits

[1] Yu, Shelly, (year). Department of Medicine Division Liver Diseases USC 'Dysregulation of GSH synthesis contributing to the pathogenesis of many pathological conditions including diabetes'. Publishing details

[2] Mitsubushi Life Sciences ( ). 'GSH RBC average decline with Age'.

[3] Sastre, J. Pallardo FV et al. ( ) 'Obesity lowers levels of Glutathione'.

[4] Alana, A, Morris MD, Liing Riyaz DDS, Patel MD et al. ( ). https://www.ncbi.nlm.nih.gov/pmc/articles/PMC3449394/

[5] Kim, YH et al. ( ). 'Induced Glutathione depletion in mice resulted in loss of behavioural Olfactory (smell) function', Buck Institute of Technology.

[6] Bergstrom, Ulrika et al. ( ) 'Inducing Glutathione depletion noted extensive damage to the Bowmans Gland – Olfactory (sense of smell) Glands', Department of Toxicology SLU, Sweden.

[7] Dr Pangrazzi, Luca ( ). 'NAC acts as an anti-oxidant and anti-inflammatory drug reducing Cytokines and Chomokenes', University of Innsbruck.

[8] Shi, Zhongcheng, Puyo, Carlos ( ). 'N Acetylcystiene to combat Covid-19', Baylor College of Medicine Houston, USA.

[9] Chen, QT et al. ( ) 'Direct and unquestionable linear relationship between blood clotting function and levels of GSH', Department of Blood Transfusion, the Second People's Hospital of Anhui Province, Hefei China.

[10] Atamna, H et al. ( ) 'Parasites use our GSH for their own protection'.

[11] Perlmutter ( ). *Grain Brain.*

[12] Loguercio, C, Piscopo, P et al. ( ) 'Relationship between Alcoholics and Cirrhotic patients and GSH depletion'.

[13] Hibberd, A.R, Howard, MA et al. ( ).

[14] Henry Spiller et al. ( ).

[15] Arab, Khelifa, Rossary, Adrien et al. ( ) 'Conjugated Linoleic Acid strongly induces Glutathione Synthesis without lipo peroxidation', German Cancer Research Center, Heidelberg Germany.

[16] Camara-Lemarroy, Carlos Rodrigo et al. (2014) 'Black Fungus'.

[17] Miravitlees, Marc (2021). 'Antibiotics – Green and Yellow Phlegm Likely to be Bacterial', Reuters.

[18] Das, Theerthanker and Simone, Martin et al. ( ) 'Glutathione can enhance Antibiotic activity', University of Sydney School of Medicine, Australia.

[19] Yildiz, D, Arik, M et al. ( ) 'NAC preferred over Cysteine in vivo experimental systems', Mustafa Kemal University Turkey.

[20] University of Michigan Health System ( ).

[21] Janson, Michael ( ). 'Glutamine Dosing', American Preventive Medical Association and the American College for Advancement in Medicine.

[22] Hanley, Jesse L. and Deville, Nancy ( ). 'Glutamine Dosing', University of Maryland Medical Centre. Livestrong.com. Daily

[23] Conte, R Castillo, B, Entranas, M et al. ( ) 'Vitamin D administered in high doses can reduce ICU admission', *Journal of Steroid Biochemistry.*

[24] Jain, Sushil, Parsanathan, R et al. ( ) 'GSH and Vitamin D Interaction. GSH stimulates Vitamin D regulatory', Louisiana State University.

[25] Alexey Polonikov( ) 'Deficiency of Glutathione as the Most Likely Cause of Serious Manifestations and Death in Covid-19', Department of Biology, Medical Genetics and Ecology and Research Institute for Genetic and Molecular Epidemiology, Kursk State Medical University, Kursk, Russian Federation. https://pubmed. ncbi.nlm.nih.gov/32463221/

[26] Horowitz, RI. Freeman, PR, Bruzzese, J. (2020) 'Efficacy of Glutathione therapy in relieving dyspnea associated with Covid-19 pneumonia'.

[27] Horowitz RI. Freeman PR, Bruzzese, J. (2020) 'Alternative prescription for a Covid-19 critical care patient'.

[28] Jackson AA, Gibson NR, Lu Y, Jahoor F. Synthesis of erythrocyte glutathione in healthy adults consuming the safe amount of dietary protein. *Am J Clin Nutr.* 2004;80(1):101–107. [PubMed] [Google Schola

[29] Glutathione Deficiency in Cardiac Patients Is Related to the Functional Status and Structural Cardiac Abnormalities Thibaud Damy, Matthias Kirsch

Risk Assessment for COVID 19 Vulnerabilities Check list

All of the below conditions can affect the patients vascular Glutathione GSH Levels

A condition where the RBC Glutathione levels are at below 1.16 - the WHO recommended minimum. A Check list including 1 of the below should trigger a blood test 3 most certainly. **Any chronic condition or long term illness** such as Cancer or treatments such as Chemotherapy should trigger a blood test so supplementation can be considered

Higher Risk Conditions

- **Glutathione Deficiency** (any reason) GSH RBC below 1.16 mmlo
- Age over 60
- Diabetes & liver disease
- Obesity
- Chronic Obesity
- Alcohol Consumption, / Alcoholic more than 3 units per day
- Pain killers
- Drug Usage Daily Dependency - Opioids, or Narcotic Analgesics
- Drug Usage Daily Dependency - Analgesics NSAIDs,Paracetamol / Ibrofen
- Drug Usage ` Daily Dependency Barbiturates
- Black Afro Caribbean / Asian hereditary
- History of Blood clotting
- Celiac or Asymptomatic Gluten-intolerant
- Any chronic condition or long term illness
- Glutathione synthetase deficiency (extremely rare 70 patients global

Lower Risk Conditions

- **Helminth Parasitic condition** previous or current condition assume some condition even asymptomatic if not treated within five years Fish or Meat eater, especially uncooked raw fish / Sushi eater.
- CLA (Conjugated Linoleic Acid Deficiency

- Patients with high Mercury amalgam Dental toxicity
- Higher Consistent Acidic Blood PH – Deficient Homeostasis
- Low Selenium Levels
- Low Vitamin C, D, & E levels

This list is not Exhaustive but would serve for primary assessment

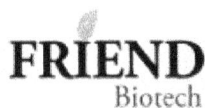

FRIEND
Biotech

Author's Note

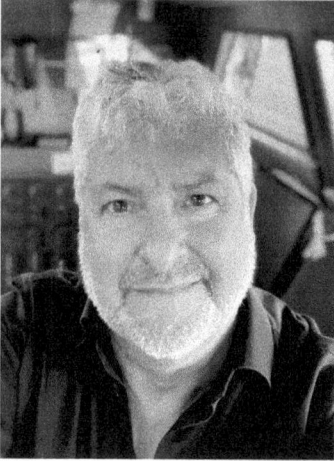

The Author, Lee Scott Friend, has studied and researched Aminos and protein structures for over 20 years after realising their importance to health. The human body cannot survive nutritionally without protein and fats. With the world's reliance on high profit based wasteful factory-farmed animal protein, given there are less than 60 years of farming topsoil left, he believes this research is the human race's most important endeavour. He runs and owns an international business group with 400 employees in 5 countries and formed Friend Biotech to research and advise on protein nutrition, medicine and production.

www.ingramcontent.com/pod-product-compliance
Lightning Source LLC
Chambersburg PA
CBHW050216270326
41914CB00003BA/433

.